THE HEART HEALTHY COOKBOOK FOR BEGINNERS

Tilda May

TABLE OF CONTENTS

4

INTRODUCTION

In our fast-paced society, maintaining a healthy lifestyle is becoming increasingly difficult. The prevalence of heart disease, which is one of the leading causes of death worldwide, lends credence to this claim. The good news is that various types of heart disease can be avoided or controlled via healthy eating habits and lifestyle choices.

This comprehensive cookbook was deliberately developed for people who want to live a heart-healthy lifestyle, making it an excellent resource for those who are just starting out. Changing your eating habits might be intimidating, which is why this book is here to assist you at every step of the process. It highlights the importance of long-term heart health and includes a number of dishes that you and your family can enjoy for decades.

This cookbook tries to dispel the idea that heart-healthy eating equals boring, unpleasant food. The recipes in this book, on the other hand, highlight the natural flavors and richness of full, nutrient-dense ingredients. By using herbs, spices, and other natural taste enhancers, you'll discover that heart-healthy meals can be just as delectable, if not more so, than the traditional diet.

This cookbook emphasizes not just the nutritional components of a heart-healthy diet, but also the importance of moderation and balance. You'll guarantee that your body gets all of the nutrients it needs by eating a range of foods and substances. You'll learn to listen to your body and make conscious food choices, which will lead to a better, more rewarding existence.

You'll learn a lot about nutrition's role in preventing and controlling heart disease as you embark on your heart-healthy path. This cookbook lays the groundwork for understanding how specific products and cooking methods can promote optimal heart health. You'll learn more about the advantages of different food groups and how to incorporate them into your diet in a balanced and tasty way.

Aside from physical health benefits, living a heart-healthy lifestyle can have a substantial impact on your emotional and mental well-being. Prioritizing self-care and investing in your health will most certainly result in increased energy, improved mood, and a greater sense of success. This cookbook is both a recipe collection and an empowering tool for helping you take control of your health and enhance your general quality of life.

As you go through the pages of this cookbook, you'll discover that a heart-healthy diet is a lifelong commitment to wellbeing, not a quick fix. And with delectable, low-sodium, and low-fat recipes at your disposal, you'll be well-equipped to make this commitment both joyful and long-lasting. Here's to enjoying a heart-healthy lifestyle for the rest of your life!

WHAT IS HEART DISEASE?

Cardiovascular disease, also referred to as heart disease, is a group of medical diseases that affect the function and appearance of the heart and blood vessels. These conditions can impair the heart's ability to efficiently circulate blood, supply oxygen and nutrients to the body's tissues, and maintain a steady beating. People sometimes use the terms "heart disease" and "cardiovascular disease" interchangeably, despite the fact that "heart disease" exclusively refers to disorders affecting the heart, whereas "cardiovascular disease" includes conditions affecting both the heart and blood arteries.

Outlined below are some of the most prevalent types of heart disease:

1. Coronary Artery Disease (CAD)

This is the most common type of heart disease. This happens when plaque, a fatty deposit buildup, builds in the arteries that feed blood to the heart muscle, causing constriction or blockage of these veins. Reduced blood circulation can cause chest pain (angina), breathing difficulty, and other symptoms. A plaque rupture can result in a blood clot that blocks the artery, resulting in a heart attack.

2. Heart Failure

Also referred to as congestive heart failure, this disorder emerges when the heart is unable to pump a sufficient amount of blood to meet the body's requisites. Heart failure can arise from various elements, including CAD, elevated blood pressure, or harm to the heart muscle from a prior heart attack.

3. Arrhythmias

These irregular heart rhythms may arise from anomalies in the heart's electrical system. Heart arrhythmias can cause the heart to beat excessively fast, too slow, or in an otherwise irregular pattern. Atrial fibrillation, bradycardia, and tachycardia are all common types of arrhythmias.

4. Heart Valve Disease

When one or more of the heart's valves malfunction, it can disrupt blood flow within the heart, leading to a condition called valvular heart disease. Valve problems can be congenital (present at birth) or develop over time due to aging, infections, or other factors.

5. Cardiomyopathy

This pertains to disorders of the heart muscle that can enfeeble the heart and impede its ability to effectively circulate blood. Several types of cardiomyopathy include dilated, hypertrophic, and restrictive cardiomyopathy.

6. Congenital Heart Defects

These are cardiac issues that exist from birth, such as a hole in the heart, faulty valves, or difficulties with the chambers of the heart. Some congenital cardiac problems are modest and may not cause symptoms, but others might be serious and necessitate early treatment.

7. Pericardial Disease

This includes issues with the pericardium, the thin sac that surrounds and protects the heart. Pericarditis (pericardium inflammation), pericardial effusion (fluid buildup around the heart), and constrictive pericarditis (pericardium thickness and scarring) can all impact how the heart works and cause symptoms such as chest pain and shortness of breath.

Causes of Heart Disease

There are many things that can lead to heart disease.

Some of the primary causes include:

1. High Blood Pressure (hypertension)

Persistently elevated blood pressure can impair the blood vessels and the heart, augmenting the likelihood of heart disease.

2. High Cholesterol

Elevated levels of low-density lipoprotein (LDL) cholesterol, also known as "bad" cholesterol, can lead to plaque buildup in the arteries, contributing to the development of CAD.

3. Smoking

Smoking has detrimental effects on blood vessels and can lead to atherosclerosis, a condition characterized by the constriction of the arteries. This makes heart disease more likely.

4. Obesity

Excessive weight places added strain on the heart and can worsen pre-existing conditions such as high blood pressure, high cholesterol, and diabetes, ultimately augmenting the chance of developing heart disease.

5. Diabetes

When blood sugar levels are too high, blood vessels and nerves can get hurt. This makes heart disease more likely.

6. Sedentary lifestyle

Physical inactivity can be a contributing factor to obesity, elevated blood pressure, and high cholesterol, thereby amplifying the hazard of heart disease.

7. Genetics and family history

A family history of heart disease can increase an individual's risk due to genetic factors and shared lifestyle habits.

Symptoms of Heart Disease

Manifestations of heart disease may differ contingent on the precise condition; nevertheless, some shared symptoms may encompass the following:

- Chest pain or discomfort (angina)
- Shortness of breath
- Dizziness or lightheadedness
- Fatigue
- Irregular heartbeat (arrhythmia)
- Swelling in the extremities (edema)
- Rapid weight gain
- Nausea or lack of appetite
- Persistent cough or wheezing

How Heart Disease is Treated

Treatment options for heart disease depend on the severity and underlying cause of the condition.

Some common treatment approaches include:

1. Medications

Various medications can be used to treat heart diseases, such as blood pressure-lowering drugs, cholesterol-lowering drugs (statins), antiplatelet medications, anticoagulants, and medications to control heart rate and rhythm.

2. Lifestyle Changes

Adopting a heart-healthy lifestyle is critical for preventing and managing heart disease. This involves eating a balanced diet, exercising regularly, keeping a healthy weight, quitting smoking, and managing stress.

3. Medical Procedures

In some cases, medical operations may be required to treat cardiac problems. Angioplasty (the practice of opening clogged arteries), stenting (the insertion of a thin mesh tube to keep an artery open), and bypass surgery (the surgical creation of a new channel for blood flow around a blocked artery) are examples.

4. Surgery

In more severe cases, heart surgery may be required, such as valve repair or replacement, heart transplant, or the implantation of a pacemaker or defibrillator to regulate the heart's electrical activity.

5. Cardiac Rehabilitation

Through exercise, education, and counseling, cardiac rehabilitation programs can assist individuals in recovering after a heart incident or procedure and adopting a heart-healthy lifestyle.

Preventive strategies and early detection are critical in lowering the risk of heart disease and improving outcomes for people who have already been diagnosed. Regular examinations with a healthcare professional, as well as monitoring and managing risk factors, can reduce the likelihood of getting heart disease or having problems greatly.

Benefits of the Heart-Healthy Eating Pattern

A diet that is conducive to heart health can notably decrease the likelihood of developing heart disease or assist in regulating pre-existing conditions.

By focusing on nutrient-dense, minimally processed foods, a heart-healthy diet provides numerous benefits for overall health and well-being:

1. Lowering Blood Pressure And Cholesterol Levels

Blood pressure and LDL ("bad") cholesterol levels can be decreased with a heart-healthy diet that prioritizes nutrient-dense foods like fruits, vegetables, whole grains, lean proteins, and healthy fats. This diminishes the probability of plaque accumulation in the arteries.

2. Reducing Inflammation And Promoting Healthy Blood Flow

Antioxidants, which are found in foods like berries, leafy greens, and nuts, can help fight inflammation. Omega-3 fatty acids, which are found in fatty fish, flaxseeds, and walnuts, can help blood flow and keep the heart healthy.

3. Supporting a Healthy Weight

A heart-healthy eating pattern, combined with regular physical activity, can help maintain a healthy weight or promote weight loss, reducing the strain on the heart and decreasing the risk of heart disease.

4. Improving Blood Sugar Control

A well-balanced diet that is abundant in fiber and low in added sugars can aid in regulating blood sugar levels, which is especially crucial for individuals with diabetes or those susceptible to developing the disorder.

5. Strengthening The Immune System

A diet full of fruits, vegetables, and whole grains gives you vitamins, minerals, and antioxidants that boost your immune system and keep you from getting sick.

6. Reducing The Risk of Other Chronic Diseases

In addition to promoting heart health, a heart-healthy eating pattern can lower the risk of other chronic diseases, such as stroke, type 2 diabetes, and certain types of cancer.

7. Enhancing Mental Health And Cognitive Function

A heart-healthy diet can also benefit mental health and cognitive function by providing essential nutrients for brain health, such as omega-3 fatty acids, antioxidants, and B vitamins.

8. Promoting Healthy Digestion

A diet that is abundant in fiber sourced from fruits, vegetables, whole grains, and legumes can promote robust digestion, avert constipation, and diminish the likelihood of gastrointestinal ailments.

9. Boosting Energy Levels And Overall Well-Being

A well-balanced, heart-healthy eating pattern can provide sustained energy throughout the day and improve overall well-being by supplying the body with the essential nutrients it needs to function optimally.

Incorporating a heart-healthy dietary pattern not only diminishes the likelihood of heart disease but also yields a plethora of supplementary health advantages.

Tips and Tricks for Following a Healthy Eating Pattern

Adopting a heart-healthy eating pattern may seem challenging at first, but with a few simple tips and tricks, you can easily make sustainable changes to your diet and enjoy the benefits of a healthier lifestyle.

1. Plan Your Meals And Snacks

Make a weekly meal and snack plan that includes a variety of nutrient-rich foods such whole grains, lean proteins, fruits, veggies, and healthy fats. This can help you make more deliberate dietary choices while decreasing the temptation to rely on harmful foods.

Create a weekly meal plan and grocery list based on heart-healthy meals that you enjoy. This will save you time and money while also ensuring that you have enough ingredients to cook healthful meals throughout the week.

2. Start with Small Changes

Rather of attempting to totally change your eating habits at once, gradually add heart-healthy changes into your diet. Small, controllable changes can add up over time and are more likely to become long-term habits.

Increase the amount of veggies in your meal, switch to whole-grain bread, or replace soda with water or herbal tea. This method will assist you in developing a heart-healthy eating pattern without feeling overwhelmed.

3. Practice Portion Control

Keeping track of portion sizes might help you avoid overeating and maintain a healthy body weight. To naturally reduce portion sizes, use smaller dishes and bowls, and pay attention to serving amounts specified on food labels. In addition, try to eat at a reasonable pace and pay attention to your body's hunger and fullness cues.

Divide your plate into pieces, with half of the plate made up of vegetables and fruits, one-fourth made up of whole grains, and the remaining quarter made up of lean proteins.

4. Cook at Home More Often

Meal preparation at home gives you more control over the ingredients and cooking methods employed, ensuring that your meals are heart-healthy. Experiment with new recipes and learn how to make your favorite dishes healthy by cutting back on sodium, saturated fats, and added sweets. This will save you money while also allowing you to gain a better grasp of the nutritional value of your meals.

5. Make Healthier Swaps

In your daily meals, swap out less healthful items for more nutritious choices. For example, instead of white rice, use brown rice or quinoa, whole wheat pasta instead of ordinary pasta, and olive oil instead of butter or margarine. These easy substitutions can greatly increase the nutritional quality of your meals without compromising flavor.

6. Limit Processed Foods and Added Sugars

Restrict your consumption of processed foods, which are frequently high in sodium, unhealthy fats, and added sugars. Instead, focus on whole, minimally processed foods, and use natural sweeteners like honey or fruit to add sweetness to your meals and snacks.

7. Experiment with Herbs and Spices

To improve flavor without relying on salt or bad fats, use a variety of herbs and spices in your culinary creations. Experiment with different flavor combinations to find your favorites, and keep a spice cabinet well-stocked to encourage heart-healthy culinary inventiveness.

8. Make Heart-Healthy Choices When Eating Out

It might be difficult to go out when attempting to eat heart-healthy, but with little forethought and awareness, you can still enjoy restaurant meals without jeopardizing your health. Select foods that are grilled, roasted, or steamed, and request sauces and dressings on the side. Avoid fried foods and high-sodium dishes, and prefer whole-grain options wherever possible.

9. Involve Family and Friends

Share your heart-healthy journey with your family and friends, and urge them to make healthier dietary choices alongside you. Cooking and eating together can provide responsibility and support while also making the experience more fun and sustainable.

10. Be Patient and Persistent

It takes time to change your eating habits, so be patient with yourself as you build a healthy nutritional pattern. Celebrate your victories while keeping in mind that setbacks are a typical part of the journey. Maintain your focus on your goals and the long-term benefits of a healthier lifestyle.

Using the following tactics, you can gradually build a heart-healthy eating pattern that is both fun and sustainable. Accept the process and remember that even little changes can have a significant influence on your overall health and well-being.

What to Eat and What to Avoid

When following a heart-healthy eating pattern, knowing which foods to include and which ones to limit or avoid is essential.

Here's a breakdown of what to eat and what to avoid, along with the health benefits and examples of each:

What to Eat:

1. Fruits and Vegetables

Fruits rich in vitamins, minerals, antioxidants, and fiber, such as apples, berries, oranges, leafy greens, tomatoes, bell peppers, broccoli, and sweet potatoes, can help lower blood pressure, reduce inflammation, and promote overall heart health. Fresh and frozen fruits are included in this category, as are dried fruits in moderation.

Make an effort to consume at least 5 servings of fruits and vegetables every day, emphasizing a variety of colors and varieties. A typical serving size is one medium-sized fruit, 1/2 cup of cooked vegetables, or 1 cup of raw leafy greens.

2. Whole Grains

Whole grains are high in fiber, which can help decrease cholesterol and keep blood sugar stable. Whole grains include barley, brown rice, quinoa, whole wheat bread, and pasta. They also include important minerals including B vitamins, iron, and magnesium, which improve heart health.

Aim for at least three servings of whole grains every day. A single serving is 1/2 cup cooked grains, one slice whole wheat bread, or one cup whole grain cereal.

3. Lean Proteins

Fish, tofu, beans, lentils, skinless poultry, and low-fat dairy products are all good sources of lean protein. Fish, particularly fatty forms like salmon, mackerel, and sardines, are high in omega-3 fatty acids, which can reduce inflammation and improve heart health. Beans and lentils help reduce blood pressure and cholesterol levels due to their high fiber and plant-based protein composition.

Aim for 2-3 portions of lean protein per day, including at least two fatty fish dishes per week. 3 ounces cooked meat or chicken, 3/4 cup cooked beans or lentils, or 1/4 cup tofu equals one serving.

4. Healthy Fats

Olive oil, almonds, seeds, and avocados are examples of healthful fats. Monounsaturated and polyunsaturated fats, which are abundant in these meals, can help lower LDL cholesterol and reduce inflammation. Nuts and seeds also include important minerals such as magnesium and vitamin E.

Attempt to consume 2-3 servings of healthy fats every day. One serving equals 1/4 cup nuts or seeds, 1/2 medium avocado, or 1 tablespoon olive oil.

What to Avoid:

1. Saturated and Trans Fats

Saturated fats, which are usually found in full-fat dairy products, fatty meats, and tropical oils such as coconut and palm oil, should be consumed in moderation. Trans fats, on the other hand, which can raise LDL cholesterol levels and increase the risk of heart disease, can be found in partially hydrogenated oils and should be avoided totally.

2. Excess Sodium

Too much sodium can cause high blood pressure, so limit your daily sodium intake to 2,300 milligrams (mg). Limit processed foods, canned goods, and restaurant meals, which are frequently rich in salt, and instead choose low-sodium or sodium-free products when they are available.

3. Added Sugars

Excessive consumption of added sugars can result in weight gain, inflammation, and elevated triglyceride levels, all of which are risk factors for heart disease. Limit consumption of sugary beverages, candies, baked goods, and other foods high in added sugars, and opt for naturally sweetened options like fruit.

4. Refined Carbohydrates

Reduce your consumption of processed carbs, which can cause blood sugar increases and weight gain. White bread, white rice, and pastries are examples of these items. Instead, choose whole-grain options that are higher in fiber and minerals.

You can build a healthy eating pattern that supports general cardiovascular health and well-being by including nutrient-dense meals and minimizing bad ones. Also, remember to keep track of your portion sizes and eat a variety of meals to ensure that you're meeting your nutritional needs.

BREAKFAST RECIPES

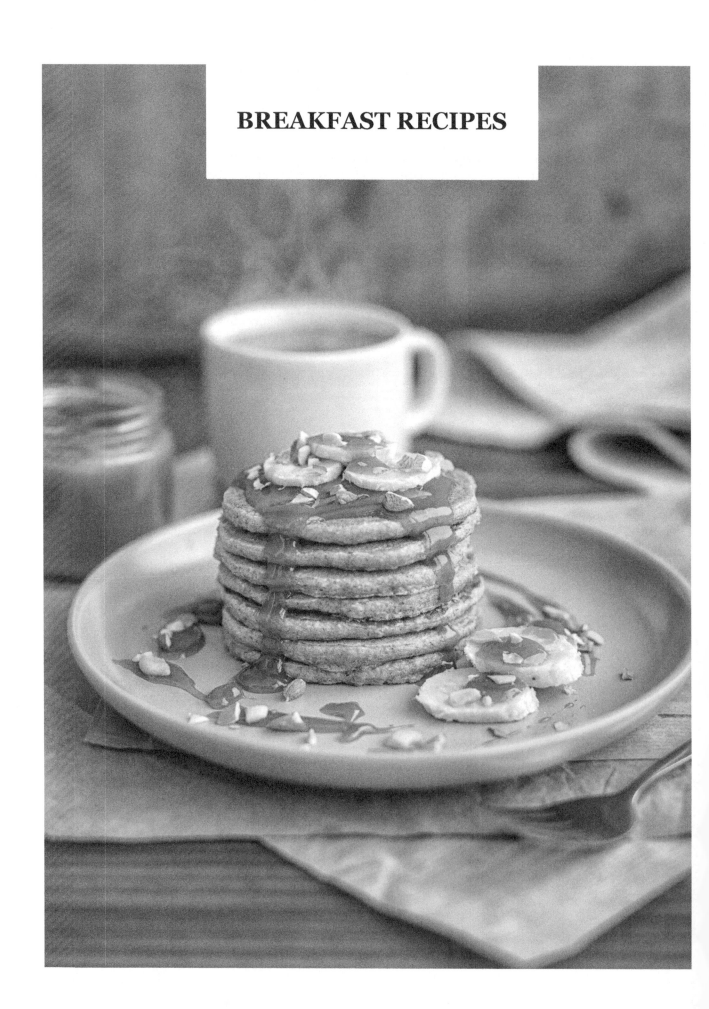

BANANA OAT PANCAKES

Ingredients:

- 1 ripe banana
- ½ cup old-fashioned oats
- ½ cup of unsweetened almond milk
- ¼ cup whole wheat flour
- ½ tsp baking powder
- ¼ tsp cinnamon
- ¼ tsp vanilla extract
- ⅛ tsp salt
- Non-stick cooking spray
- ¼ cup fresh blueberries (optional)

Instructions:

1. Combine banana, oats, almond milk, whole wheat flour, baking powder, cinnamon, vanilla extract, and salt in a blender. Blend until smooth.
2. Before cooking, preheat a non-stick skillet over medium heat and lightly coat it with non-stick cooking spray.
3. Pour ¼ cup of batter onto the skillet for each pancake. If using blueberries, sprinkle a few onto each pancake.
4. Let the ingredients cook for 2 to 3 minutes, or until bubbles form on the surface. Then, flip them over and cook for another 1 to 2 minutes, or until they turn golden brown.
5. Serve right away with your favorite toppings, like honey or fresh fruit.

Nutritional Values (per serving):

Calories: 245 | Fat: 3.5g | Saturated Fat: 0.5g | Cholesterol: 0mg | Sodium: 175mg | Carbohydrates: 47g | Fiber: 7g | Sugar: 9g | Protein: 8g

SPINACH AND MUSHROOM EGG WHITE SCRAMBLE

Ingredients:

- 4 large egg whites
- 1 cup baby spinach, chopped
- ½ cup mushrooms, sliced
- ¼ cup diced onion
- ¼ cup diced red bell pepper
- ¼ cup low-sodium feta cheese, crumbled
- ¼ tsp garlic powder
- ¼ tsp black pepper
- ¼ tsp dried basil
- Non-stick cooking spray

Instructions:

1. In a medium mixing bowl, combine the egg whites, garlic powder, black pepper, and dried basil. Place aside.
2. Coat a nonstick skillet with nonstick cooking spray and heat on medium.
3. Heat the onions and bell peppers in a pan. Cook for about 3-4 minutes, or until they begin to soften.
4. When the mushrooms are cooked, return them to the pan and cook for another 3-4 minutes.
5. Toss the spinach into the skillet after the other ingredients have completed cooking. Cook for 1-2 minutes, or until the spinach has wilted.
6. Pour the egg white mixture over the cooked veggies in the skillet. Cook, stirring periodically, until the egg whites are fully cooked and no longer runny.
7. Remove from the pan and top with the low-sodium feta cheese.
8. Serve immediately with whole-grain toast or fresh fruit on the side.

Nutritional Values (per serving):

Calories: 164 | Fat: 4g | Saturated Fat: 2g | Cholesterol: 10mg | Sodium: 290mg | Carbohydrates: 11g | Fiber: 3g | Sugar: 4g | Protein: 20g

OVERNIGHT CHIA PUDDING

Ingredients:

- ½ cup of unsweetened almond milk
- ½ cup plain Greek yogurt
- ¼ cup chia seeds
- ½ tsp vanilla extract
- ½ tsp honey
- ½ cup mixed berries (fresh or frozen)
- 2 tbsp chopped nuts (e.g., almonds, walnuts, or pecans)

Instructions:

1. Take a small bowl and whisk together the almond milk, Greek yogurt, chia seeds, vanilla extract, and honey until they are well combined.
2. Evenly distribute the mixture between two little jars or containers, then secure the lids.
3. Once you've mixed all the ingredients together, cover the bowl and put it in the fridge for at least 4 hours or overnight so the chia seeds can soak up the liquid and make the pudding thicker.
4. Top each pudding with mixed berries and chopped nuts when ready to serve.

Nutritional Values (per serving):

Calories: 250 | Fat: 13g | Saturated Fat: 1g | Cholesterol: 5mg | Sodium: 115mg | Carbohydrates: 24g | Fiber: 11g | Sugar: 8g | Protein: 12g

AVOCADO AND TOMATO TOAST

Ingredients:

- 2 slices whole-grain bread
- ½ ripe avocado
- ½ cup cherry tomatoes, halved
- ¼ tsp garlic powder
- ¼ tsp black pepper
- ¼ tsp red pepper flakes (optional)
- ¼ tsp dried basil
- ¼ tsp lemon juice

Instructions:

1. Toast the bread pieces until they are as crisp as you like.
2. Take a small bowl and mash the avocado in it using a fork. Add garlic powder, black pepper, and lemon juice to the mashed avocado and mix until well combined.
3. On the toast slices, evenly distribute the mashed avocado.

4. Top each slice with halved cherry tomatoes and sprinkle with dried basil and red pepper flakes.
5. Serve immediately.

Nutritional Values (per serving):

Calories: 278 | Fat: 14g | Saturated Fat: 2g | Cholesterol: 0mg | Sodium: 260mg | Carbohydrates: 33g | Fiber: 9g | Sugar: 5g | Protein: 9g

APPLE CINNAMON QUINOA BREAKFAST BOWL

Ingredients:

- ¼ cup dry quinoa
- ½ cup water
- ¼ cup unsweetened almond milk
- ½ apple, diced
- ¼ tsp cinnamon
- ¼ tsp vanilla extract
- 1 tbsp chopped nuts (e.g., almonds, walnuts, or pecans)
- 1 tbsp dried cranberries

Instructions:

1. Start by heating up some water in a small saucepan until it boils.
2. When the water has boiled, add the quinoa and turn down the heat. When the quinoa has absorbed all the water and is fully cooked, add the water to the pot with the quinoa.
3. Cover the pot and let the mixture simmer for about 12 to 15 minutes.
4. Stir in the almond milk, diced apple, cinnamon, and vanilla extract, and cook for another 3-4 minutes until heated through.
5. Divide the quinoa mixture between two bowls and top with chopped nuts and dried cranberries.
6. Serve immediately.

Nutritional Values (per serving):

Calories: 235 | Fat: 7g | Saturated Fat: 1g | Cholesterol: omg | Sodium: 40mg | Carbohydrates: 38g | Fiber: 5g | Sugar: 9g | Protein: 6g

VEGGIE AND EGG BREAKFAST BURRITO

Ingredients:

- 2 whole wheat tortillas
- 4 large egg whites
- ¼ cup diced onion
- ¼ cup diced bell pepper
- ¼ cup diced tomato
- ¼ cup canned low-sodium black beans, rinsed and drained
- ¼ tsp ground cumin
- ¼ tsp black pepper
- ¼ cup shredded low-fat cheddar cheese
- Non-stick cooking spray

Instructions:

1. In a medium mixing bowl, combine the egg whites, cumin, and black pepper. Place aside.
2. Spray a nonstick pan lightly with nonstick cooking spray and heat it to medium.
3. Heat the onions and bell peppers in a pan. Cook for about 3-4 minutes, or until they begin to soften.
4. When everything is hot, add the tomatoes and black beans, mix well, and cook for another 2-3 minutes.
5. Pour the egg white mixture over the cooked veggies in the skillet. Cook, stirring periodically, until the egg whites are fully cooked and no longer runny.
6. Microwave the tortillas for 15-20 seconds or cook them in a dry pan over low heat for 1-2 minutes per side.
7. Evenly distribute the egg and veggie mixture between the two tortillas and top with shredded low-fat cheddar cheese.
8. To make a burrito, roll the dough up and fold the sides in. Serve immediately.

Nutritional Values (per serving):

Calories: 285 | Fat: 6g | Saturated Fat: 2g | Cholesterol: 5mg | Sodium: 430mg | Carbohydrates: 38g | Fiber: 8g | Sugar: 4g | Protein: 20g

GREEK YOGURT AND BERRY PARFAIT

Ingredients:

- ½ cup mixed berries (fresh or frozen)
- ¼ cup low-fat granola
- 1 cup plain non-fat Greek yogurt
- ½ tsp honey

Instructions:

1. Put half of the Greek yogurt in a glass or bowl. Then add half of the mixed berries and half of the granola.
2. Repeat the layers with the remaining Greek yogurt, mixed berries, and granola.
3. Pour the honey on top, and serve it right away.

Nutritional Values (per serving):

Calories: 265 | Fat: 3g | Saturated Fat: 0g | Cholesterol: 5mg | Sodium: 80mg | Carbohydrates: 38g | Fiber: 5g | Sugar: 22g | Protein: 23g

PEANUT BUTTER AND BANANA SMOOTHIE

Ingredients:

- 1 ripe banana, sliced and frozen
- ½ cup of unsweetened almond milk
- ¼ cup plain non-fat Greek yogurt
- 1 tbsp natural peanut butter
- ½ tsp honey
- ¼ tsp vanilla extract
- ¼ cup ice (optional)

Instructions:

1. In a blender, combine the frozen banana slices, almond milk, Greek yogurt, peanut butter, honey, vanilla extract,

and ice (if using). Mix until creamy and smooth.

2. Put the smoothie in two glasses right away and serve.

Nutritional Values (per serving):

Calories: 210 | Fat: 8g | Saturated Fat: 1g | Cholesterol: 0mg | Sodium: 135mg | Carbohydrates: 27g | Fiber: 3g | Sugar: 15g | Protein: 10g

VEGETABLE OMELET

Ingredients:

- 4 large egg whites
- ¼ cup diced bell pepper
- ¼ cup diced onion
- ¼ cup chopped mushrooms
- ¼ cup diced tomato
- ¼ cup chopped baby spinach
- ¼ tsp garlic powder
- ¼ tsp black pepper
- ¼ cup shredded low-fat cheddar cheese
- Non-stick cooking spray

Instructions:

1. In a medium-sized mixing bowl, combine the garlic powder, black pepper, and egg whites. Set the mixture aside to be used later. Next, heat a nonstick pan over medium heat. Lightly coat the skillet with nonstick cooking spray. Add the onions and bell peppers to the skillet and sauté for 3-4 minutes, or until they begin to soften. After 3-4 minutes, add the mushrooms to the skillet and simmer for another 3-4 minutes, or until soft.

2. Cook the tomatoes and baby spinach for 1-2 minutes, stirring periodically, or until the spinach wilts.

3. When the vegetables are done, pour the egg white mixture in the skillet over them. When the sides start to solidify but the middle is still a bit fluid, the mixture is ready, which takes about 3 to 4 minutes.

4. Cover one side of the omelet with low-fat cheddar cheese crumbles. The remaining half should be neatly wrapped over the cheese.

5. Cook for another 1-2 minutes, or until the cheese melts and the omelet is done.

6. Cut the omelet in half and serve immediately.

Nutritional Values (per serving):

Calories: 140 | Fat: 2g | Saturated Fat: 1g | Cholesterol: 5mg | Sodium: 280mg | Carbohydrates: 11g | Fiber: 3g | Sugar: 4g | Protein: 18g

BERRY OATMEAL

Ingredients:

- 1 cup old-fashioned oats
- 2 cups water
- ¼ tsp cinnamon
- ¼ tsp vanilla extract
- ½ cup mixed berries (fresh or frozen)
- 1 tbsp chopped nuts (e.g., almonds, walnuts, or pecans)
- ½ tsp honey

Instructions:

1. Bring the water to a boil in a medium-sized pot. Put the oats in the pot, and turn the heat down to low. Simmer the oats for 5-7 minutes, occasionally stirring, until they become tender and have absorbed all the water.
2. Stir in the cinnamon and vanilla extract.
3. Separate the oats evenly into two bowls and add a mixture of berries, chopped nuts, and a slight drizzle of honey on top of each.
4. Serve immediately.

Nutritional Values (per serving):

Calories: 230 | Fat: 6g | Saturated Fat: 1g | Cholesterol: 0mg | Sodium: 10mg | Carbohydrates: 38g | Fiber: 6g | Sugar: 8g | Protein: 7g

TROPICAL GREEN SMOOTHIE

Ingredients:

- 1 cup baby spinach

- ½ cup frozen pineapple chunks
- ½ cup frozen mango chunks
- ½ banana, sliced and frozen
- 1 cup unsweetened almond milk
- ¼ cup plain non-fat Greek yogurt
- ½ tsp honey

Instructions:

1. In a blender, combine the baby spinach, frozen pineapple chunks, frozen mango chunks, frozen banana slices, almond milk, Greek yogurt, and honey. Blend until smooth and creamy.
2. Once the smoothie is blended to your desired consistency, divide it evenly into two glasses and serve immediately.

Nutritional Values (per serving):

Calories: 150 | Fat: 2g | Saturated Fat: 0g | Cholesterol: 0mg | Sodium: 120mg | Carbohydrates: 30g | Fiber: 4g | Sugar: 21g | Protein: 7g

COTTAGE CHEESE AND FRUIT BOWL

Ingredients:

- 1 cup low-fat cottage cheese
- ½ cup mixed fruit (e.g., berries, diced peaches, or pineapple)
- ¼ cup low-fat granola
- 1 tbsp chopped nuts (e.g., almonds, walnuts, or pecans)
- ½ tsp honey

Instructions:

1. Put the oats in the pot, and turn the heat down to low.
2. Top each bowl with mixed fruit, low-fat granola, chopped nuts, and a drizzle of honey.
3. Serve immediately.

Nutritional Values (per serving):

Calories: 255 | Fat: 6g | Saturated Fat: 1g | Cholesterol: 10mg | Sodium: 380mg | Carbohydrates: 32g | Fiber: 3g | Sugar: 20g | Protein: 20g

MULTIGRAIN WAFFLES WITH FRUIT

Ingredients:

- 2 frozen multigrain waffles
- ½ cup mixed berries (fresh or frozen)
- ¼ cup plain non-fat Greek yogurt
- ½ tsp honey
- ¼ tsp ground cinnamon

Instructions:

1. Toast the frozen multigrain waffles according to the package directions.
2. Mix the Greek yogurt, honey, and cinnamon in a small bowl.
3. Top each waffle with half of the yogurt mixture and a portion of mixed berries.
4. Serve immediately.

Nutritional Values (per serving):

Calories: 240 | Fat: 7g | Saturated Fat: 1g | Cholesterol: 0mg | Sodium: 380mg | Carbohydrates: 36g | Fiber: 5g | Sugar: 11g | Protein: 10g

ALMOND BUTTER AND APPLE RICE CAKES

Ingredients:

- 2 brown rice cakes
- 2 tbsp natural almond butter
- ½ apple, thinly sliced
- ¼ tsp ground cinnamon

Instructions:

1. Spread 1 tbsp of almond butter onto each rice cake.

2. Place the apple slices on top of the almond butter, making sure there are equal amounts on each rice cake.
3. Dust the apple slices with cinnamon powder.

Nutritional Values (per serving):

Calories: 235 | Fat: 12g | Saturated Fat: 1g | Cholesterol: 0mg | Sodium: 45mg | Carbohydrates: 28g | Fiber: 4g | Sugar: 9g | Protein: 6g

SPINACH, TOMATO, AND MOZZARELLA FRITTATA

Ingredients:

- 4 large egg whites
- ½ cup of baby spinach, chopped
- ½ cup cherry tomatoes, halved
- ¼ cup shredded low-fat mozzarella cheese
- ¼ tsp garlic powder
- ¼ tsp black pepper
- ¼ tsp dried basil
- Non-stick cooking spray

Instructions:

1. In a medium-sized mixing bowl, combine the egg whites, garlic powder, black pepper, and dried basil until thoroughly combined. Please do not use the bowl.
2. Preheat the oven to 375°F (190°C) before you begin cooking.
3. Heat an oven-safe nonstick skillet over medium heat, spraying it lightly with nonstick cooking spray.
4. Place the baby spinach in the pan and simmer for one to two minutes, or until soft.
5. Cook for 1-2 minutes more after adding the cherry tomatoes.
6. Pour the egg white mixture into the skillet with the spinach and cook for 3 to 4 minutes, or until the sides are set but the middle is still fluid.
7. Sprinkle the frittata with shredded low-fat mozzarella cheese.
8. Bake for 8 to 10 minutes, or until the cheese has melted and the frittata is done.

9. Remove the frittata from the oven, let it cool for a minute, and then cut it in two. Serve immediately.

Nutritional Values (per serving):

Calories: 125 | Fat: 2g | Saturated Fat: 1g | Cholesterol: 5mg | Sodium: 270mg | Carbohydrates: 6g | Fiber: 1g | Sugar: 3g | Protein:18g

SMOKED SALMON AND AVOCADO RICE CAKE

Ingredients:

- 2 brown rice cakes
- ¼ cup mashed avocado
- ¼ tsp black pepper
- ¼ tsp lemon juice
- 2 oz smoked salmon
- ¼ cup cucumber, thinly sliced
- 1 tbsp capers (optional)

Instructions:

1. In a small bowl, mix together the mashed avocado, black pepper, and lemon juice.
2. On the rice cakes, evenly distribute the avocado mixture.
3. Each rice cake should have smoked salmon and cucumber slices on top.
4. Optionally, sprinkle capers over the top.
5. Serve immediately.

Nutritional Values (per serving):

Calories: 250 | Fat: 12g | Saturated Fat: 2g | Cholesterol: 10mg | Sodium: 720mg | Carbohydrates: 23g | Fiber: 3g | Sugar: 1g | Protein: 14g

TURKEY SAUSAGE AND VEGGIE SCRAMBLE

Ingredients:

- 2 turkey sausage links, cooked and sliced
- ½ cup chopped bell pepper
- ½ cup chopped onion
- ½ cup chopped mushrooms
- ½ cup chopped zucchini
- 4 large egg whites
- ¼ tsp garlic powder
- ¼ tsp black pepper
- Non-stick cooking spray

Instructions:

1. In a medium mixing bowl, combine the egg whites, garlic powder, and black pepper. Place aside.
2. Lightly coat a nonstick skillet with cooking spray and heat it over medium heat.
3. Place the onions and peppers in a pan. Cook for about 3-4 minutes, or until they begin to soften.
4. Cook for an additional 3-4 minutes, or until the mushrooms and zucchini are tender.
5. Stir in the cooked turkey sausage slices and simmer for 1-2 minutes, or until completely heated.
6. Pour the egg-white mixture over the cooked veggies and sausage in the skillet. Cook for 3-4 minutes, occasionally lifting the sides to enable the uncooked egg to seep below. Cook the omelet until it is completely cooked and no longer moist.
7. Divide the scramble between two dishes and serve immediately.

Nutritional Values (per serving):

Calories: 200 | Fat: 6g | Saturated Fat: 1g | Cholesterol: 35mg | Sodium: 450mg | Carbohydrates: 15g | Fiber: 3g | Sugar: 5g | Protein: 22g

CHIA PUDDING WITH FRUIT

Ingredients:

- ¼ cup chia seeds
- 1 cup unsweetened almond milk
- ½ tsp vanilla extract
- ½ tsp honey
- ½ cup mixed fruit (e.g., berries, diced peaches, or pineapple)

Instructions:

1. Combine the chia seeds, almond milk, vanilla extract, and honey in a small bowl or jar.
2. Cover the bowl or jar and place it in the refrigerator overnight, or for a minimum of 4 hours, until the chia seeds have absorbed the liquid and the mixture has attained the consistency of pudding.
3. When the pudding is ready to be served, divide it between two bowls or jars. Top each with a portion of mixed fruit and serve immediately.

Nutritional Values (per serving):

Calories: 180 | Fat: 8g | Saturated Fat: 1g | Cholesterol: 0mg | Sodium: 100mg | Carbohydrates: 21g | Fiber: 10g | Sugar: 9g | Protein: 6g

GREEK YOGURT WITH GRANOLA AND BERRIES

Ingredients:

- 1 cup non-fat plain Greek yogurt
- ¼ cup low-fat granola
- ½ cup mixed berries (e.g., blueberries, raspberries, or strawberries)
- 1 tsp honey (optional)

Instructions:

1. Divide the Greek yogurt between two bowls.
2. Top each bowl with half of the granola and mixed berries.
3. Optionally, drizzle each bowl with honey before serving.

Nutritional Values (per serving):

Calories: 195 | Fat: 2g | Saturated Fat: 0g | Cholesterol: 5mg | Sodium: 60mg | Carbohydrates: 30g | Fiber: 3g | Sugar: 18g | Protein: 16g

AVOCADO AND EGG TOAST

Ingredients:

- 2 slices whole-grain bread
- ½ avocado, mashed
- ¼ tsp black pepper
- ¼ tsp lemon juice
- 2 large eggs
- Non-stick cooking spray

Instructions:

1. Toast the whole-grain bread slices.
2. Mix the mashed avocado, black pepper, and lemon juice in a small bowl.
3. Heat a nonstick skillet over medium-high heat. Apply a thin layer of nonstick cooking spray to the skillet. Gently break the eggs and add them to the pan, cooking until they reach your preferred level of doneness.
4. Spread the avocado mixture onto the toast slices, then top each with a cooked egg.
5. Serve immediately.

Nutritional Values (per serving):

Calories: 320 | Fat: 18g | Saturated Fat: 3g | Cholesterol: 185mg | Sodium: 310mg | Carbohydrates: 27g | Fiber: 7g | Sugar: 4g | Protein: 15g

PINEAPPLE, BANANA, AND SPINACH SMOOTHIE

Ingredients:

- 1 cup fresh or frozen pineapple chunks
- 1 ripe banana
- 1 cup baby spinach
- ½ cup unsweetened almond milk
- ½ cup non-fat plain Greek yogurt
- 1 tbsp honey (optional)

Instructions:

1. Blend the pineapple, banana, spinach, almond milk, Greek yogurt, and honey (if desired) together until the mixture is smooth.
2. Immediately after blending, transfer the contents of the smoothie into two glasses and serve promptly.

Nutritional Values (per serving):

Calories: 190 | Fat: 1g | Saturated Fat: 0g | Cholesterol: 0mg | Sodium: 110mg | Carbohydrates: 40g | Fiber: 4g | Sugar: 27g | Protein: 8g

QUINOA AND BERRY BREAKFAST BOWL

Ingredients:

- ½ cup cooked quinoa
- ½ cup mixed berries (e.g., blueberries, raspberries, or strawberries)
- ¼ cup non-fat plain Greek yogurt
- 1 tbsp chopped nuts (e.g., almonds, walnuts, or pecans)
- 1 tsp honey (optional)

Instructions:

1. Divide the cooked quinoa between two bowls.
2. Greek yogurt, chopped nuts, and half of the mixed berries should be placed on top of each bowl.
3. Optionally, drizzle each bowl with honey before serving.

Nutritional Values (per serving):

Calories: 210 | Fat: 4g | Saturated Fat: 0g | Cholesterol: 0mg | Sodium: 30mg | Carbohydrates: 34g | Fiber: 5g | Sugar: 11g | Protein: 11g

GREEN DETOX SMOOTHIE

Ingredients:

- 1 cup baby spinach
- ½ cucumber chopped

- ½ green apple chopped
- ½ cup fresh or frozen pineapple chunks
- ½ cup unsweetened almond milk
- ½ cup water
- ½ cup ice (optional)

Instructions:

1. In a blender, combine the spinach, cucumber, green apple, pineapple, almond milk, water, and ice (if using). Blend until smooth.
2. Blend the ingredients until smooth, then pour the smoothie into two glasses and serve immediately.

Nutritional Values (per serving):

Calories: 80 | Fat: 1g | Saturated Fat: 0g | Cholesterol: 0mg | Sodium: 70mg | Carbohydrates: 17g | Fiber: 3g | Sugar: 11g | Protein: 2g

VEGGIE AND HUMMUS WRAP

Ingredients:

- 2 whole-grain tortillas
- ¼ cup hummus
- ½ cup shredded lettuce
- ½ cup chopped bell pepper
- ½ cup chopped cucumber
- ½ cup grated carrot

Instructions:

1. Lay the whole-grain tortillas on a flat surface.
2. Spread half of the hummus on each tortilla.
3. Top each tortilla with half of the shredded lettuce, bell pepper, cucumber, and grated carrot.
4. Roll the tortillas firmly, folding in the sides as you proceed.
5. Each wrap should be cut in half and served right away.

Nutritional Values (per serving):

Calories: 220 | Fat: 7g | Saturated Fat: 1g | Cholesterol: 0mg | Sodium: 400mg |

Carbohydrates: 34g | Fiber: 7g | Sugar: 5g | Protein: 8g

COTTAGE CHEESE AND FRUIT BOWL

Ingredients:

- 1 cup low-fat cottage cheese
- ½ cup mixed fruit (e.g., berries, diced peaches, or pineapple)
- 1 tbsp chopped nuts (e.g., almonds, walnuts, or pecans)
- 1 tsp honey (optional)

Instructions:

1. The cottage cheese should be split between two bowls.
2. Top each bowl with half of the mixed fruit and chopped nuts.
3. Optionally, drizzle each bowl with honey before serving.

Nutritional Values (per serving):

Calories: 180 | Fat: 4g | Saturated Fat: 1g | Cholesterol: 5mg | Sodium: 400mg | Carbohydrates: 20g | Fiber: 2g | Sugar: 15g | Protein: 16g

SNACK RECIPES

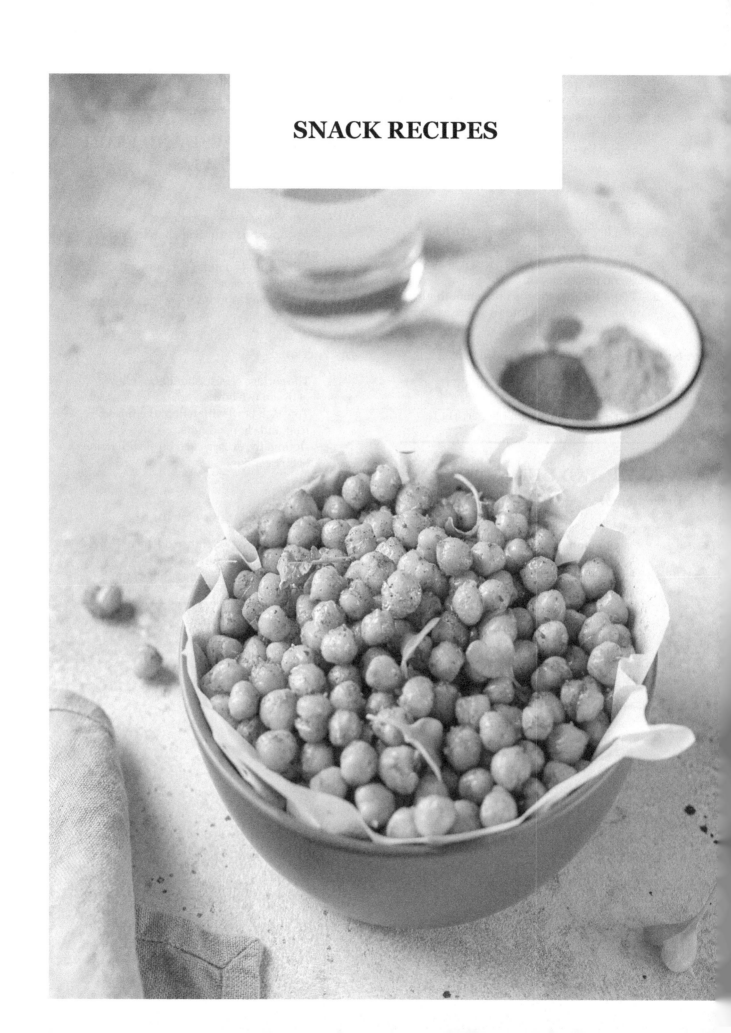

SPICY ROASTED CHICKPEAS

Ingredients:

- 1 (15 oz) can of chickpeas, drained, rinsed, and patted dry
- 1 tbsp olive oil
- ¼ tsp paprika
- ¼ tsp garlic powder
- ¼ tsp cayenne pepper
- ¼ tsp salt

Instructions:

1. Set the oven's temperature to 400°F (200°C). Use parchment paper to line a baking sheet.
2. Combine the chickpeas, olive oil, paprika, garlic powder, cayenne pepper, and salt in a mixing bowl.
3. Arrange the chickpeas in a single layer on the prepared baking sheet.
4. Bake for 30-35 minutes, or until crispy and golden brown, shaking the pan halfway through.
5. Allow the chickpeas to cool slightly before serving. Keep leftovers in a container that does not allow air to enter.

Nutritional Values (per serving):

Calories: 130 | Fat: 5g | Saturated Fat: 0.5g | Cholesterol: 0mg | Sodium: 250mg | Carbohydrates: 17g | Fiber: 5g | Sugar: 3g | Protein: 6g

GREEK YOGURT RANCH DIP WITH VEGGIES

Ingredients:

- 1 cup non-fat plain Greek yogurt
- 1 tbsp dry ranch dressing mix
- 2 cups mixed vegetables (e.g., baby carrots, celery sticks, cucumber slices, or cherry tomatoes)

Instructions:

1. Mix the Greek yogurt and dry ranch dressing mix together in a small bowl.
2. Divide the Greek yogurt ranch dip and mixed vegetables between two plates.

3. Serve immediately.

Nutritional Values (per serving):

Calories: 110 | Fat: 0g | Saturated Fat: 0g | Cholesterol: 5mg | Sodium: 430mg | Carbohydrates: 14g | Fiber: 3g | Sugar: 7g | Protein: 12g

APPLE SLICES WITH ALMOND BUTTER

Ingredients:

- 1 large apple, cored and sliced
- 2 tbsp almond butter

Instructions:

1. Divide the apple slices between two plates.
2. Serve each plate with 1 tablespoon of almond butter for dipping.

Nutritional Values (per serving):

Calories: 190 | Fat: 10g | Saturated Fat: 1g | Cholesterol: 0mg | Sodium: 0mg | Carbohydrates: 24g | Fiber: 5g | Sugar: 17g | Protein: 4g

MINI CAPRESE SKEWERS

Ingredients:

- 10 cherry tomatoes
- 10 small fresh mozzarella balls
- 10 fresh basil leaves
- 1 tbsp balsamic glaze

Instructions:

1. Thread a cherry tomato, mozzarella ball, and basil leaf onto each of the 10 small skewers.
2. Before serving, put the skewers on a plate and drizzle them with balsamic glaze.

Nutritional Values (per serving):

Calories: 150 | Fat: 9g | Saturated Fat: 5g | Cholesterol: 30mg | Sodium: 200mg | Carbohydrates: 9g | Fiber: 1g | Sugar: 7g | Protein: 9g

CELERY STICKS WITH CREAM CHEESE AND EVERYTHING BAGEL SEASONING

Ingredients:

- 4 celery stalks cut into 3-inch sticks
- ¼ cup low-fat cream cheese
- 1 tbsp everything bagel seasoning

Instructions:

1. Fill the celery sticks with cream cheese.
2. Everything bagel seasoning should be put on the celery sticks that have been filled.
3. The celery sticks should be divided between two plates and served.

Nutritional Values (per serving):

Calories: 80| Fat: 4g | Saturated Fat: 2.5g | Cholesterol: 15mg | Sodium: 320mg | Carbohydrates: 6g | Fiber: 1g | Sugar: 2g | Protein: 4g

AVOCADO-STUFFED CHERRY TOMATOES

Ingredients:

- 12 cherry tomatoes
- 1 ripe avocado, mashed
- ¼ tsp garlic powder
- ¼ tsp black pepper
- ¼ tsp lemon juice

Instructions:

1. Slice the tops of the cherry tomatoes and carefully scoop out the insides with a small spoon.

2. Mix the mashed avocado, garlic powder, black pepper, and lemon juice in a small bowl.
3. Use a small spoon or a piping bag to put the avocado mixture into the cherry tomatoes.
4. The stuffed cherry tomatoes should be divided between two plates and served.

Nutritional Values (per serving):

Calories: 130 | Fat: 10g | Saturated Fat: 1.5g | Cholesterol: 0mg | Sodium: 25mg | Carbohydrates: 10g | Fiber: 4g | Sugar: 4g | Protein: 2g

CUCUMBER SLICES WITH HUMMUS

Ingredients:

- 1 large cucumber, sliced
- ¼ cup hummus

Instructions:

1. Divide the cucumber slices between two plates.
2. Serve each plate with 2 tablespoons of hummus for dipping.

Nutritional Values (per serving):

Calories: 80 | Fat: 4g | Saturated Fat: 0.5g | Cholesterol: 0mg | Sodium: 180mg | Carbohydrates: 10g | Fiber: 2g | Sugar: 2g | Protein: 4g

ANTS ON A LOG

Ingredients:

- 4 celery stalks cut into 3-inch sticks
- 2 tbsp peanut butter
- 2 tbsp raisins

Instructions:

1. Fill the celery sticks with peanut butter.

2. Press the raisins into the peanut butter on each celery stick.
3. Divide the ants on a log between two plates and serve.

Nutritional Values (per serving):

Calories: 170 | Fat: 9g | Saturated Fat: 2g | Cholesterol: 0mg | Sodium: 115mg | Carbohydrates: 20g | Fiber: 2g | Sugar: 12g | Protein: 5g

EASY EDAMAME

Ingredients:

- 1 cup frozen shelled edamame
- ¼ tsp salt
- ¼ tsp black pepper

Instructions:

1. Cook the edamame according to the package instructions, usually by boiling or steaming for 3-5 minutes.
2. After draining the edamame, sprinkle with salt and black pepper to taste.
3. Divide the edamame between two plates and serve warm.

Nutritional Values (per serving):

Calories: 100 | Fat: 4g | Saturated Fat: 0.5g | Cholesterol: 0mg | Sodium: 310mg | Carbohydrates: 9g | Fiber: 4g | Sugar: 2g | Protein: 8g

PEANUT BUTTER AND CHOCOLATE RICE CAKES

Ingredients:

- 2 brown rice cakes
- 2 tbsp peanut butter
- 2 tsp chocolate chips

Instructions:

1. On each rice cake, spread 1 tablespoon of peanut butter.
2. Sprinkle each rice cake with 1 teaspoon of chocolate chips.
3. Serve immediately.

Nutritional Values (per serving):

Calories: 210 | Fat: 11g | Saturated Fat: 2.5g | Cholesterol: 0mg | Sodium: 75mg | Carbohydrates: 23g | Fiber: 1g | Sugar: 8g | Protein: 5g

SPINACH AND ARTICHOKE DIP

Ingredients:

- ½ cup non-fat plain Greek yogurt
- ½ cup canned artichoke hearts, drained and chopped
- ½ cup chopped spinach (fresh or thawed frozen)
- ¼ cup grated Parmesan cheese
- ¼ tsp garlic powder
- ¼ tsp black pepper
- Whole grain crackers or raw veggies for serving

Instructions:

1. Combine Greek yogurt, artichoke hearts, spinach, Parmesan cheese, garlic powder, and black pepper in a medium-sized bowl.
2. Serve the dip with whole grain crackers or raw veggies.

Nutritional Values (per serving):

Calories: 100 | Fat: 3g | Saturated Fat: 1.5g | Cholesterol: 10mg | Sodium: 320mg | Carbohydrates: 7g | Fiber: 1g | Sugar: 3g | Protein: 11g

FRUIT KABOBS WITH HONEY-YOGURT DRIP

Ingredients:

- 1 cup mixed fruit (e.g., berries, grapes, pineapple, or kiwi)
- ½ cup non-fat plain Greek yogurt
- 1 tbsp honey

Instructions:

1. Thread the mixed fruit onto 4 skewers.
2. Mix the Greek yogurt and honey in a small bowl.
3. Divide the fruit kabobs and honey-yogurt dip between two plates and serve.

Nutritional Values (per serving):

Calories: 120 | Fat: 0g | Saturated Fat: 0g | Cholesterol: 0mg | Sodium: 25mg | Carbohydrates: 26g | Fiber: 2g | Sugar: 22g | Protein: 6g

SLICED TURKEY AND CHEESE ROLL-UPS

Ingredients:

- 4 slices low-sodium deli turkey
- 2 slices reduced-fat Swiss cheese, halved
- 4 large lettuce leaves

Instructions:

1. Lay a lettuce leaf on a flat surface.
2. Place a slice of deli turkey on the lettuce leaf.
3. Top the turkey with a half slice of Swiss cheese.
4. Tightly roll the lettuce leaf, tucking the sides in as you go.
5. Repeat steps 1-4 with the remaining ingredients.
6. Divide the turkey and cheese roll-ups between two plates and serve.

Nutritional Values (per serving):

Calories: 100 | Fat: 4g | Saturated Fat: 2g | Cholesterol: 30mg | Sodium: 380mg |

Carbohydrates: 2g | Fiber: 0g | Sugar: 1g | Protein: 14g

POPCORN WITH NUTRITIONAL YEAST

Ingredients:

- 3 cups air-popped popcorn
- 1 tbsp olive oil
- 2 tbsp nutritional yeast
- ¼ tsp salt

Instructions:

1. Drizzle the olive oil over the popcorn and toss to coat.
2. Sprinkle the nutritional yeast and salt over the popcorn, and toss again to distribute the seasonings evenly.
3. Divide the popcorn between two bowls and serve.

Nutritional Values (per serving):

Calories: 120 | Fat: 7g | Saturated Fat: 1g | Cholesterol: 0mg | Sodium: 300mg | Carbohydrates: 10g | Fiber: 2g | Sugar: 0g | Protein: 4g

BELL PEPPER NACHOS

Ingredients:

- 1 large bell pepper, sliced into thin strips
- ¼ cup black beans rinsed and drained
- ¼ cup shredded reduced-fat cheddar cheese
- 2 tbsp diced tomatoes
- 2 tbsp diced avocado

Instructions:

1. Set the oven's temperature to 400°F (200°C). Cover a baking sheet with parchment paper.
2. Put one layer of bell pepper slices on the baking sheet.

3. Top the bell pepper slices with black beans and shredded cheddar cheese.
4. For 5–7 minutes, bake the cheese until it melts and starts to bubble.
5. When it comes out of the oven, put diced avocado and tomato on top.
6. The nachos with bell peppers should be split between two plates and served.

Nutritional Values (per serving):

Calories: 130 | Fat: 6g | Saturated Fat: 2g | Cholesterol: 10mg | Sodium: 180mg | Carbohydrates: 13g | Fiber: 4g | Sugar: 3g | Protein: 8g

VEGGIE PINWHEELS

Ingredients:

- 1 large whole wheat tortilla
- 2 tbsp reduced-fat cream cheese
- ½ cup mixed vegetables (e.g., shredded carrots, cucumber, or bell pepper)

Instructions:

1. Spread the cream cheese on the whole wheat tortilla.
2. Arrange the mixed vegetables on the tortilla.
3. Roll the tortilla tightly and slice it into 1-inch pinwheels.
4. Place two pinwheels on each of two plates and serve.

Nutritional Values (per serving):

Calories: 110 | Fat: 3g | Saturated Fat: 1g | Cholesterol: 10mg | Sodium: 260mg | Carbohydrates: 16g | Fiber: 2g | Sugar: 2g | Protein: 4g

FROZEN YOGURT BARK

Ingredients:

- 1 cup non-fat plain Greek yogurt
- 1 tbsp honey
- ¼ cup mixed berries
- 1 tbsp chopped nuts (e.g., almonds, walnuts, or pecans)

Instructions:

1. Line a baking sheet with parchment paper.
2. Mix the Greek yogurt and honey in a small bowl.
3. Evenly spread the yogurt mixture onto the prepared baking sheet in a thin layer.
4. Scatter the mixed berries and chopped nuts over the yogurt layer.
5. Place in the freezer for a minimum of 2 hours or until the mixture becomes firm.
6. Split the frozen yogurt bark into pieces and put them on two plates in an even way. Serve immediately.

Nutritional Values (per serving):

Calories: 150 | Fat: 4g | Saturated Fat: 0.5g |Cholesterol: 0mg | Sodium: 45mg | Carbohydrates: 18g | Fiber: 1g | Sugar: 15g | Protein: 12g

CHOCOLATE BANANA BITES

Ingredients:

- 1 large banana, sliced
- 2 tbsp dark chocolate chips
- 1 tsp coconut oil

Instructions:

1. Line a baking sheet or plate with parchment paper.
2. In a small microwave-safe bowl, combine the dark chocolate chips and coconut oil. Microwave the chocolate in 15-second increments, stirring after each interval, until it has melted and smooth. Place each banana slice on the prepared dish and dip it into the melted chocolate, letting the excess drip off.
3. Place the chocolate-covered banana slices in the freezer for at least 1 hour, or until solid.
4. Divide the frozen banana bites between two dishes and serve.

Nutritional Values (per serving):

Calories: 150 | Fat: 7g | Saturated Fat: 5g | Cholesterol: 0mg | Sodium: 0mg | Carbohydrates: 23g | Fiber: 2g | Sugar: 15g | Protein: 1g

Nutritional Values (per serving):

Calories: 150 | Fat: 6g | Saturated Fat: 3g | Cholesterol: 15mg | Sodium: 250mg | Carbohydrates: 14g | Fiber: 2g | Sugar: 2g | Protein: 9g

SMOKED SALMON AND CREAM CHEESE CUCUMBER BITES

Ingredients:

- 1 large cucumber, sliced
- 4 oz smoked salmon, cut into small pieces
- ¼ cup reduced-fat cream cheese
- 1 tbsp chopped fresh dill

Instructions:

1. Top each cucumber slice with a small piece of smoked salmon.
2. Dollop a small amount of cream cheese onto each smoked salmon-topped cucumber slice.
3. Sprinkle a little fresh dill on each bite of cucumber.
4. Serve the cucumber bites by dividing them between two plates.

Nutritional Values (per serving):

Calories: 100 | Fat: 4g | Saturated Fat: 2g | Cholesterol: 20mg | Sodium: 430mg | Carbohydrates: 4g | Fiber: 1g | Sugar: 2g | Protein: 11g

CHEESE AND CRACKERS

Ingredients:

- 2 oz reduced-fat cheddar cheese, sliced
- 10 whole grain crackers

Instructions:

1. Divide the cheese slices and whole-grain crackers between two plates.
2. Serve immediately.

MEAT RECIPES

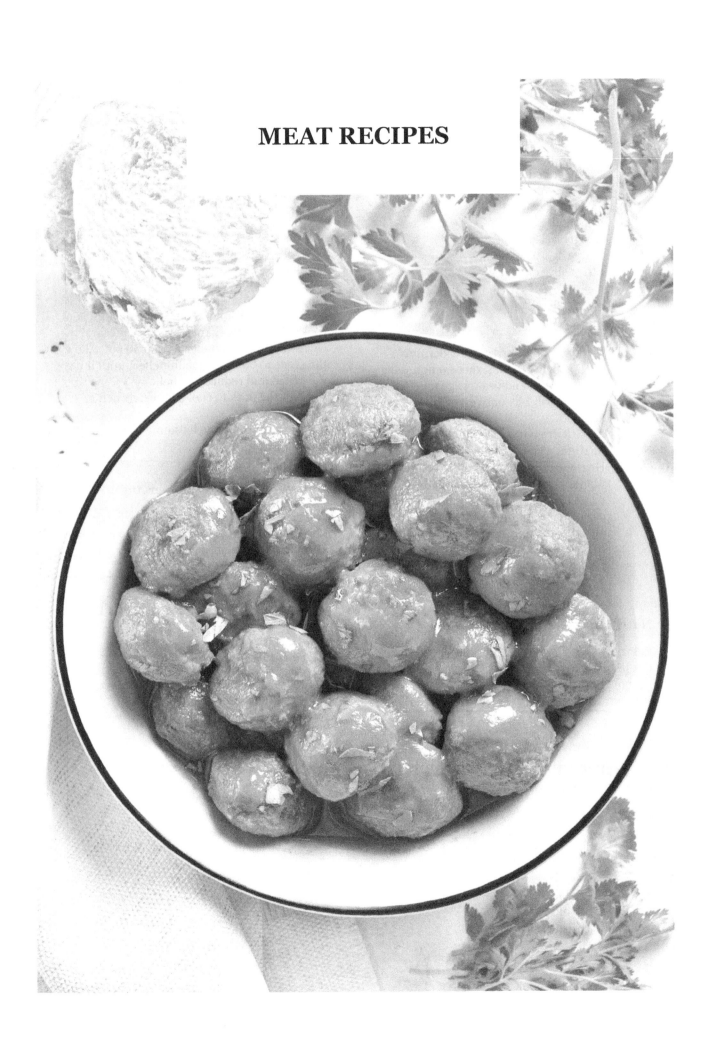

TURKEY MEATBALLS

Ingredients:

- ½ lb lean ground turkey
- ¼ cup whole wheat breadcrumbs
- ¼ cup grated Parmesan cheese
- ¼ cup chopped fresh parsley
- ¼ tsp garlic powder
- ¼ tsp salt
- ¼ tsp black pepper
- 1 large egg, beaten
- 1 tbsp olive oil

Instructions:

1. Mix the ground turkey, breadcrumbs, chopped mushrooms, diced onion, salt, black pepper, and beaten egg together in a large bowl. Mix until everything is well blended.
2. Make 8 even-sized meatballs from the mixture.
3. Heat the olive oil on medium heat in a non-stick pan. Add the meatballs to the pan and cook for 8-10 minutes, flipping occasionally, until they are browned on all sides and fully cooked.
4. Serve the turkey meatballs with your favorite marinara sauce or on top of whole wheat spaghetti.

Nutritional Values (per serving):

Calories: 250 | Fat: 13g | Saturated Fat: 4g | Cholesterol: 105mg | Sodium: 460mg | Carbohydrates: 8g | Fiber: 1g | Sugar: 1g | Protein: 24g

PORK TENDERLOIN WITH BALSAMIC GLAZE

Ingredients:

- ½ lb pork tenderloin, trimmed of excess fat
- ¼ tsp salt
- ¼ tsp black pepper
- 1 tbsp olive oil
- ¼ cup balsamic vinegar
- ¼ cup low-sodium chicken broth
- 1 tbsp honey

Instructions:

1. Set the oven to 375°F (190°C) and turn it on.
2. Season the pork tenderloin to taste with salt and black pepper.
3. Heat the olive oil in a medium-high oven-safe pan. Cook the pork tenderloin for 2-3 minutes on each side, or until browned.
4. Place the skillet in the oven for about 20 minutes, or until the pork is done.
5. Make the balsamic glaze while the pork is cooking by blending the balsamic vinegar, chicken stock, and honey in a small pot. Allow the sauce to boil over medium heat until it has thickened and reduced by half.
6. Allow the pork to cool completely before slicing.
7. To serve, drizzle the balsamic glaze over the sliced pork.

Nutritional Values (per serving):

Calories: 280 | Fat: 12g | Saturated Fat: 2.5g | Cholesterol: 80mg | Sodium: 420mg | Carbohydrates: 12g | Fiber: 0g | Sugar: 10g | Protein: 29g

BEEF STIR-FRY WITH BROCCOLI

Ingredients:

- ½ lb lean beef sirloin, thinly sliced
- ¼ tsp salt
- ¼ tsp black pepper
- 1 tbsp olive oil
- 1 cup broccoli florets
- ¼ cup low-sodium soy sauce
- ¼ cup water
- ½ tbsp cornstarch
- ½ tbsp honey
- ½ tsp minced garlic
- ½ tsp grated fresh ginger

Instructions:

1. Season the meat slices with black pepper and salt.
2. Heat olive oil in a large nonstick skillet over medium-high heat. Cook the meat in the skillet for 2-3 minutes on each side, or until it is browned. Remove the steak from the pan and set it aside.
3. To the same skillet, add the broccoli florets and sauté for 4 to 5 minutes, or until soft but still crisp.
4. Whisk together the soy sauce, water, cornstarch, honey, garlic, and ginger in a small bowl. Drizzle the sauce evenly over the broccoli in the pan after adding it to the pan, and simmer for another 2 to 3 minutes, or until the sauce has thickened to the desired consistency.
5. Return the steak to the skillet and toss it in with the remaining ingredients to incorporate. Allow the mixture to cook for an additional 2-3 minutes, or until well heated.
6. Serve the beef stir-fry on two dishes with brown rice or quinoa.

Nutritional Values (per serving):

Calories: 340 | Fat: 14g | Saturated Fat: 3g | Cholesterol: 80mg | Sodium: 820mg | Carbohydrates: 14g | Fiber: 2g | Sugar: 7g | Protein: 36g

BAKED CHICKEN FAJITA STUFFED PEPPERS

Ingredients:

- 2 large bell peppers, halved and seeded
- ½ lb boneless, skinless chicken breasts, cooked and shredded
- ¼ cup diced onion
- ¼ cup diced tomato
- ¼ cup low-sodium black beans, rinsed and drained
- ¼ cup frozen corn, thawed
- ¼ tsp chili powder
- ¼ tsp cumin
- ¼ tsp paprika
- ¼ tsp garlic powder
- ¼ tsp salt
- ¼ cup shredded reduced-fat cheddar cheese

Instructions:

1. Set the oven's temperature to 375°F (190°C). Using parchment paper, line a baking sheet.
2. In a large mixing bowl, combine the shredded chicken, onion, tomato, black beans, corn, cumin, paprika, garlic powder, and salt.
3. Fill each bell pepper half halfway with the chicken mixture, pressing firmly.
4. Arrange the stuffed peppers on the previously prepared baking sheet and bake for 25-30 minutes, or until they reach the required softness.
5. When the peppers are done, take them from the oven and top with shredded cheddar cheese. Return the casserole to the oven for another 2-3 minutes to properly melt the cheese.
6. When the stuffed peppers are done, divide them equally between two dishes and serve.

Nutritional Values (per serving):

Calories: 290 | Fat: 6g | Saturated Fat: 2g | Cholesterol: 85mg | Sodium: 520mg | Carbohydrates: 23g | Fiber: 6g| Sugar: 7g | Protein: 36g

GREEK-STYLE GRILLED CHICKEN

Ingredients:

- 2 boneless, skinless chicken breasts
- ¼ cup plain low-fat Greek yogurt
- ¼ cup olive oil
- ¼ tsp garlic powder
- ¼ tsp dried oregano
- ¼ tsp dried thyme
- ¼ tsp salt
- ¼ tsp black pepper
- ½ lemon, juiced

Instructions:

1. 1. Combine Greek yogurt, olive oil, garlic powder, dried oregano, dried thyme, salt, black pepper, and lemon juice in a shallow plate.
2. 2. Add the chicken breasts to the marinade and turn them over to coat well. Refrigerate the dish, covered with a

lid or plastic wrap, for at least 30 minutes or up to 2 hours to chill and marinate.

3. 3. Preheat the grill or grill pan to high heat before grilling. Remove the chicken from the marinade and shake off any excess marinade to ensure that it is not overly moist.

4. 4. Grill the chicken for 6-7 minutes on each side until it is cooked through and the internal temperature reaches 165°F (74°C).

5. 5. Before serving, remove the chicken from the grill and let it aside for a few minutes to rest.

Nutritional Values (per serving):

Calories: 250 | Fat: 13g | Saturated Fat: 2g | Cholesterol: 85mg | Sodium: 380mg | Carbohydrates: 2g | Fiber: 0g | Sugar: 1g | Protein: 28g

BALSAMIC-GLAZED PORK CHOPS

Ingredients:

- 2 boneless pork chops, about 1/2 lb
- ¼ tsp salt
- ¼ tsp black pepper
- 1 tbsp olive oil
- ¼ cup balsamic vinegar
- 1 tbsp honey
- ¼ tsp dried rosemary

Instructions:

1. Add salt and black pepper to the pork chops.

2. In a pan, heat the olive oil over medium heat. Cook each side of the pork chops for only 4 to 5 minutes, as they should be fully cooked in this amount of time.

3. Whisk the balsamic vinegar, honey, and dried rosemary together in a small bowl.

4. The balsamic glaze should be applied to the pork chops after they have finished cooking. Cook the sauce for another 1 to 2 minutes, stirring it often, until it thickens and coats all of the pork chops.

5. After cooking, remove the pork chops from the pan and allow them to rest for a few minutes before serving.

Nutritional Values (per serving):

Calories: 280 | Fat: 14g | Saturated Fat: 3.5g | Cholesterol: 75mg | Sodium: 400mg | Carbohydrates: 10g | Fiber: 0g | Sugar: 9g | Protein: 28g

BEEF AND VEGETABLE STIR-FRY

Ingredients:

- ½ lb lean beef sirloin, thinly sliced
- ¼ tsp salt
- ¼ tsp black pepper
- 1 tbsp olive oil
- 1 cup mixed vegetables (such as bell peppers, carrots, and snap peas)
- ¼ cup low-sodium soy sauce
- ¼ cup water
- ½ tbsp cornstarch
- ½ tbsp honey
- ½ tsp minced garlic
- ½ tsp grated fresh ginger

Instructions:

1. Season the meat slices with black pepper and salt.
2. Heat the olive oil in a large nonstick skillet over medium heat. Cook the beef in the pan for 2-3 minutes on each side, or until it turns brown. Remove the steak from the pan and set it aside.
3. Add the vegetable mixture to the skillet and heat for 4 to 5 minutes, or until the veggies are soft but still crunchy.
4. Using a whisk, properly combine and stir the soy sauce, water, cornstarch, honey, garlic, and ginger in a small bowl. Pour the sauce over the veggies in the skillet after mixing together the sauce ingredients. Cook for another 2 to 3 minutes, or until the sauce has thickened to your liking.
5. Return the beef to the skillet, along with the veggies, and thoroughly incorporate all

ingredients to ensure they are completely combined. Cook the mixture for another 2-3 minutes, or until it is thoroughly cooked and reaches the desired temperature.
6. Serve the meat and vegetable stir-fry on two dishes with brown rice or quinoa.

Nutritional Values (per serving):

Calories: 340 | Fat: 14g | Saturated Fat: 3g | Cholesterol: 80mg | Sodium: 820mg | Carbohydrates: 16g | Fiber: 3g | Sugar: 8g | Protein: 36g

SLOW COOKER BEEF STEW

Ingredients:

- ½ lb lean beef stew meat cubed
- ¼ tsp salt
- ¼ tsp black pepper
- ¼ tsp garlic powder
- ¼ tsp onion powder
- ¼ tsp paprika
- 1 tbsp olive oil
- 1 cup low-sodium beef broth
- ½ cup diced tomatoes
- 1 cup diced potatoes
- 1 cup sliced carrots
- 1 cup chopped celery
- ½ cup diced onion

Instructions:

1. Sprinkle salt, black pepper, garlic powder, onion powder, and paprika over the beef stew meat.
2. In a nonstick skillet, heat the olive oil over medium heat until it is heated. Cook the seasoned beef in the skillet for 4 to 5 minutes, or until it is brown on all sides.
3. Using a spoon or spatula, transfer the browned beef from the skillet to the slow cooker. Combine the beef broth, diced tomatoes, diced potatoes, sliced carrots, chopped celery, and diced onion in a large mixing bowl.
4. Set the slow cooker to low heat and cook the beef and veggies for 7-8 hours, or set it to high heat and cook for 4-5 hours, until the beef is soft and the vegetables are well cooked.

5. To serve, divide the beef stew between two bowls.

Nutritional Values (per serving):

Calories: 350 | Fat: 12g | Saturated Fat: 3g | Cholesterol: 75mg | Sodium: 520mg | Carbohydrates: 27g | Fiber: 5g | Sugar: 6g | Protein: 30g

SHEET PAN SAUSAGE AND VEGETABLES

Ingredients:

- ½ lb turkey sausage, sliced
- 1 cup diced bell peppers
- 1 cup diced zucchini
- 1 cup diced red onion
- 1 cup cherry tomatoes
- 1 tbsp olive oil
- ¼ tsp salt
- ¼ tsp black pepper
- ¼ tsp garlic powder
- ¼ tsp dried basil
- ¼ tsp dried oregano

Instructions:

1. Set the oven's temperature to 400°F (200°C). Using parchment paper, line a baking sheet.
2. Combine the sliced turkey sausage, diced bell peppers, diced zucchini, diced red onion, and cherry tomatoes in a large mixing dish. Drizzle the dish with olive oil and season with salt, black pepper, garlic powder, dried basil, and dried oregano. To coat, toss with a fork.
3. Arrange the sausage and veggies on the prepared baking sheet in an even layer, making sure they are spread out in a single layer.
4. Place the baking sheet in the oven for 20-25 minutes, or until the veggies have softened and the sausage has browned to your liking.
5. Divide the sausage and vegetables between two dishes with a serving spoon and serve immediately.

Nutritional Values (per serving):

Calories: 320 | Fat: 16g | Saturated Fat: 3.5g |
Cholesterol: 85mg | Sodium: 810mg |
Carbohydrates: 19g | Fiber: 4g | Sugar: 9g |
Protein: 26g

CHICKEN AND RICE STUFFED BELL PEPPERS

Ingredients:

- 2 large bell peppers, halved and seeded
- ½ lb boneless, skinless chicken breasts, cooked and shredded
- 1 cup cooked brown rice
- ¼ cup diced onion
- ¼ cup diced tomato
- ¼ cup low-sodium black beans, rinsed and drained
- ¼ cup frozen corn, thawed
- ¼ tsp salt
- ¼ tsp black pepper
- ¼ tsp cumin
- ¼ tsp paprika
- ¼ tsp garlic powder
- ¼ cup shredded reduced-fat cheddar cheese

Instructions:

1. Set the oven's temperature to 375°F (190°C). Using parchment paper, line a baking sheet.
2. In a large mixing bowl, combine the cooked brown rice, shredded chicken, onion, tomato, black beans, corn, salt, black pepper, cumin, garlic powder, and paprika.
3. Stuff each half of a bell pepper with the chicken-rice mixture, pushing hard to fill the peppers.
4. Place the stuffed peppers on the prepared baking sheet and bake for 25-30 minutes, or until the peppers attain the desired amount of softness.
5. Remove the peppers from the oven and evenly sprinkle each with shredded cheddar cheese. Return the dish to the oven for another 2-3 minutes, or until the cheese is completely melted.
6. Divide the stuffed peppers evenly between two dishes with a spatula or serving spoon and serve hot.

Nutritional Values (per serving):

Calories: 310 | Fat: 6g | Saturated Fat: 2g |
Cholesterol: 85mg | Sodium: 540mg |
Carbohydrates: 33g | Fiber: 6g | Sugar: 7g |
Protein: 29g

SPAGHETTI SQUASH BOLOGNESE

Ingredients:

- 1 medium spaghetti squash, halved and seeded
- 1 tbsp olive oil
- ½ lb lean ground beef
- ¼ cup diced onion
- ¼ cup diced carrot
- ¼ cup diced celery
- ¼ tsp salt
- ¼ tsp black pepper
- 1 cup low-sodium marinara sauce
- ¼ cup grated Parmesan cheese

Instructions:

1. Set the oven's temperature to 400°F (200°C). Using parchment paper, line a baking sheet.
2. Brush the cut sides of the spaghetti squash with olive oil before placing them face down on the prepared baking sheet. Cook the squash for 40-45 minutes, or until it is soft enough to shred easily with a fork.
3. In the meantime, heat a nonstick pan over medium heat. Season with salt and black pepper then add the ground beef, onion, carrot, and celery. Break up the beef with a spoon while cooking it with the veggies for 8-10 minutes, or until the beef is brown and the vegetables are tender.
4. Stir the marinara sauce into the skillet with the beef and vegetables. Cook for another 5 minutes, or until the mixture is thoroughly cooked and reaches the desired temperature.
5. Remove the spaghetti squash from the oven and allow it to cool before handling. Scrape the inside of the squash with a fork to shred it into spaghetti-like threads.

6. Serve the spaghetti squash on two dishes, topped with the Bolognese beef sauce. Serve with grated Parmesan cheese on top.

Nutritional Values (per serving):

Calories: 420 | Fat: 21g | Saturated Fat: 7g | Cholesterol: 80mg | Sodium: 690mg | Carbohydrates: 32g | Fiber: 7g | Sugar: 13g | Protein: 27g

GARLIC HERB PORK TENDERLOIN

Ingredients:

- ½ lb pork tenderloin
- ¼ tsp salt
- ¼ tsp black pepper
- 1 tbsp olive oil
- 2 cloves garlic, minced
- ½ tsp dried rosemary
- ½ tsp dried thyme
- ½ tsp dried sage

Instructions:

1. Set the oven's temperature to 375°F (190°C). Line a baking sheet with parchment paper.
2. Season the pork tenderloin with salt and black pepper. Mix the minced garlic, dried rosemary, dried thyme, olive oil, and dried sage together in a small bowl.
3. Coat the entire pork tenderloin with the mixture, using your hands to press it down and help it stick to the meat.
4. Put the seasoned pork tenderloin on the prepared baking sheet and cook it in the oven for approximately 25-30 minutes or until it is thoroughly cooked.
5. Once the pork tenderloin is done cooking, remove it from the oven, and allow it to rest for a few minutes before slicing it.

Nutritional Values (per serving):

Calories: 250 | Fat: 14g | Saturated Fat: 3.5g | Cholesterol: 85mg | Sodium: 380mg |

Carbohydrates: 1g | Fiber: 0g | Sugar: 0g | Protein: 27g

CHICKEN AND BROCCOLI STIR-FRY

Ingredients:

- ½ lb boneless, skinless chicken breasts, thinly sliced
- ¼ tsp salt
- ¼ tsp black pepper
- 1 tbsp olive oil
- 1 cup chopped broccoli
- ¼ cup low-sodium chicken broth
- ¼ cup low-sodium soy sauce
- ½ tbsp cornstarch
- ½ tbsp honey
- ½ tsp minced garlic
- ½ tsp grated fresh ginger

Instructions:

1. Season the chicken slices with black pepper and salt.
2. Heat olive oil in a large nonstick skillet over medium heat. Cook the chicken in the pan for 2 to 3 minutes per side, or until the surface browns. Arrange the chicken on a plate. Remove it from the pan.
3. When the broccoli is cooked but still crunchy, add the chopped broccoli to the same pan and cook for 4 to 5 minutes more.
4. Combine the chicken broth, soy sauce, honey, garlic, and ginger in a small bowl. Combine the ingredients thoroughly. When the sauce has thickened, pour it over the broccoli and boil for 2 to 3 minutes more. Return the cooked chicken to the pan and toss everything together. Cook the mixture for another 2-3 minutes, or until it is thoroughly cooked and reaches the desired temperature.
5. Serve the chicken and broccoli stir-fry on two dishes with brown rice or quinoa.

Nutritional Values (per serving):

Calories: 300 | Fat: 10g | Saturated Fat: 1.5g | Cholesterol: 85mg | Sodium: 860mg | Carbohydrates: 16g | Fiber: 2g | Sugar: 8g | Protein: 34g

TURKEY MEATBALL SUBS

Ingredients:

- ½ lb lean ground turkey
- ¼ cup whole wheat breadcrumbs
- ¼ cup grated Parmesan cheese
- ¼ cup finely chopped fresh parsley
- ¼ tsp salt
- ¼ tsp black pepper
- ¼ tsp garlic powder
- 1 large egg, beaten
- 1 tbsp olive oil
- 1 cup low-sodium marinara sauce
- 2 whole wheat sub rolls, split
- ½ cup shredded reduced-fat mozzarella cheese

Instructions:

1. To begin, combine the ground turkey, breadcrumbs, grated Parmesan cheese, chopped parsley, salt, black pepper, garlic powder, and beaten egg in a large mixing bowl. Combine and incorporate all of the ingredients thoroughly until properly combined.
2. Form the mixture into 1-1.5-inch-diameter meatballs.
3. Melt the butter in a large nonstick skillet over medium heat. Cook the meatballs in the pan for about 6-7 minutes, turning regularly, until browned on all sides.
4. Distribute the marinara sauce evenly over the meatballs in the skillet, then cover with a lid. Reduce the heat to a moderate simmer and cook the mixture for 15-20 minutes, or until the meatballs are fully cooked.
5. Preheat the oven to broil. On a baking sheet, arrange the divided sub rolls.
6. Evenly divide the meatballs and sauce between the two sub rolls. Shredded mozzarella cheese should be sprinkled on top of the meatballs and sauce in each sub roll.
7. Broil the cheese for two to three minutes, or until it is bubbly and melted. Serve immediately after removing from the oven.

Nutritional Values (per serving):

Calories: 540 | Fat: 22g | Saturated Fat: 7g | Cholesterol: 130mg | Sodium: 980mg | Carbohydrates: 48g | Fiber: 6g | Sugar: 9g | Protein: 37g

GRILLED PORTOBELLO MUSHROOM BURGERS

Ingredients:

- 2 large portobello mushroom caps, cleaned and stems removed
- 1 tbsp olive oil
- ¼ tsp salt
- ¼ tsp black pepper
- ¼ tsp garlic powder
- ¼ tsp dried basil
- 2 whole wheat hamburger buns, split
- ½ cup sliced red onion
- ½ cup sliced tomato
- ¼ cup baby spinach leaves

Instructions:

1. Preheat the grill to medium-high heat.
2. Salt, black pepper, garlic powder, and dried basil are added to the portobello mushroom caps that have been brushed with olive oil.
3. Place the mushroom caps on the grill and cook for approximately 4-5 minutes per side, or until they are tender and have a slightly charred appearance.
4. Split the hamburger buns in half and toast them on the grill for 1 to 2 minutes until they are lightly browned.
5. To assemble the burgers, place a grilled portobello mushroom cap on the bottom half of each bun. Add sliced red onion, sliced tomato, and baby spinach leaves on top of the grilled portobello mushroom cap on each bun.

Nutritional Values (per serving):

Calories: 280 | Fat: 11g | Saturated Fat: 1.5g | Cholesterol: 0mg | Sodium: 500mg | Carbohydrates: 37g | Fiber: 6g | Sugar: 6g | Protein: 10g

GREEK CHICKEN PITA POCKETS

Ingredients:

- ½ lb boneless, skinless chicken breasts, thinly sliced
- ¼ tsp salt
- ¼ tsp black pepper
- ¼ tsp dried oregano
- 1 tbsp olive oil
- 2 whole wheat pita pockets, halved
- ½ cup chopped cucumber
- ½ cup chopped tomato
- ¼ cup sliced red onion
- ¼ cup crumbled feta cheese

Instructions:

1. Season the chicken slices with salt, black pepper, and dried oregano.
2. Heat up the olive oil in a non-stick pan over medium-high heat. Place the chicken in the pan and cook for 2 to 3 minutes per side, or until the chicken is fully cooked and browned. Put the chicken on a plate after removing it from the pan.
3. Warm the pita pockets for a few seconds in the oven or microwave to make them easier to work with.
4. Stuff each pita pocket half with cooked chicken, chopped cucumber, chopped tomato, sliced red onion, and crumbled feta cheese.
5. Serve the pita pockets with a side of Greek yogurt or tzatziki sauce for dipping, if desired.

Nutritional Values (per serving):

Calories: 380 | Fat: 12g | Saturated Fat: 4g | Cholesterol: 85mg | Sodium: 720mg | Carbohydrates: 38g | Fiber: 6g | Sugar: 4g | Protein: 31g

PHILLY CHEESESTEAK STUFFED PEPPERS

Ingredients:

- 2 large green bell peppers, halved and seeded
- ½ lb lean beef sirloin, thinly sliced
- ¼ tsp salt
- ¼ tsp black pepper
- 1 tbsp olive oil
- ½ cup sliced onion
- ½ cup sliced mushrooms
- ¼ cup shredded reduced-fat provolone cheese

Instructions:

1. Set the oven's temperature to 375°F (190°C). Cover a baking sheet with parchment paper.
2. Sprinkle salt and black pepper over the beef sirloin slices to season them.
3. Heat the olive oil in a non-stick pan over medium heat. Put the beef, onion, and mushrooms in the pan. Cook the beef and vegetables for 4-5 minutes, occasionally stirring until the beef is browned and the vegetables are tender.
4. Stuff the beef and vegetable mixture into each half of the bell pepper. Shred some provolone cheese and put it on top.
5. On the baking sheet previously prepared, bake the stuffed peppers for around 20-25 minutes until the cheese has melted and is bubbly.
6. Divide the Philly cheesesteak stuffed peppers between two plates and serve.

Nutritional Values (per serving):

Calories: 330 | Fat: 15g | Saturated Fat: 5g | Cholesterol: 75mg | Sodium: 590mg | Carbohydrates: 14g | Fiber: 3g | Sugar: 6g | Protein: 33g

BBQ-PULLED CHICKEN SANDWICHES

Ingredients:

- ½ lb boneless, skinless chicken breasts
- ¼ tsp salt
- ¼ tsp black pepper
- ½ cup low-sodium chicken broth

- ½ cup BBQ sauce, divided
- 2 whole wheat hamburger buns, split
- ½ cup coleslaw

Instructions:

1. Season the chicken breasts with a sprinkle of salt and black pepper.
2. Add the chicken, chicken broth, and 1/4 cup of BBQ sauce to a slow cooker. Slow-cook the chicken for 4-5 hours on low or 2-3 hours on high until it is fully cooked and can be effortlessly shredded with a fork.
3. After removing the chicken from the slow cooker, use two forks to shred the chicken apart. Stir in the remaining 1/4 cup of BBQ sauce, making sure it is evenly distributed throughout the shredded chicken.
4. Divide the shredded BBQ chicken between the two split hamburger buns. Top each sandwich with coleslaw and serve.

Nutritional Values (per serving):

Calories: 380 | Fat: 6g | Saturated Fat: 1g | Cholesterol: 80mg | Sodium: 810mg | Carbohydrates: 46g | Fiber: 4g | Sugar: 19g | Protein: 34g

BEEF AND VEGETABLE-STIR FRY

Ingredients:

- ½ lb lean beef sirloin, thinly sliced
- ¼ tsp salt
- ¼ tsp black pepper
- 1 tbsp olive oil
- 1 cup chopped bell peppers (any color)
- 1 cup chopped zucchini
- ¼ cup low-sodium beef broth
- ¼ cup low-sodium soy sauce
- ½ tbsp cornstarch
- ½ tbsp honey
- ½ tsp minced garlic
- ½ tsp grated fresh ginger

Instructions:

1. Season the meat slices with black pepper and salt.
2. Melt the butter in a large nonstick skillet over medium heat. Cook the beef in the pan for about 2 to 3 minutes per side, or until it is browned. Remove the steak from the skillet and set it aside.
3. Add the bell peppers and zucchini to the same pan. Cook the beef and vegetables for another 4 to 5 minutes, or until the vegetables are cooked but still crunchy.
4. Whisk together the beef stock, soy sauce, cornstarch, honey, garlic, and ginger in a small mixing bowl until fully blended. Add the small mixing bowl mixture to the pan with the vegetables and beef. Cook for another 2 to 3 minutes, or until the sauce has thickened to the desired consistency.
5. Return the cooked meat to the skillet and toss in the vegetables and sauce until completely incorporated. Cook the mixture for another 2-3 minutes, or until it is thoroughly cooked and reaches the desired temperature.
6. Serve the meat and vegetable stir-fry on two dishes with brown rice or quinoa.

Nutritional Values (per serving):

Calories: 330 | Fat: 12g | Saturated Fat: 2.5g | Cholesterol: 60mg | Sodium: 860mg | Carbohydrates: 19g | Fiber: 2g | Sugar: 9g | Protein: 33g

TURKEY TACO WRAPS

Ingredients:

- ½ lb lean ground turkey
- ¼ tsp salt
- ¼ tsp black pepper
- ¼ tsp cumin
- ¼ tsp paprika
- ¼ tsp garlic powder
- ¼ cup low-sodium chicken broth
- 6 large iceberg or butter lettuce leaves
- ½ cup chopped tomato
- ¼ cup shredded reduced-fat cheddar cheese
- ¼ cup salsa

Instructions:

1. The ground turkey should be cooked in a nonstick skillet over medium heat while being broken up with a spoon. Add salt, black pepper, cumin, paprika, and garlic powder to taste. Cook until browned and fully cooked through.
2. Add the chicken broth to the pan and cook the mixture for an additional 2-3 minutes, or until the liquid has evaporated and the ingredients are well combined.
3. Incorporate the turkey mixture into lettuce leaves. Top with chopped tomato, shredded cheddar cheese, and salsa.
4. Take the lettuce leaves and use them to wrap around the filling, ensuring that the filling is completely covered by the lettuce. Serve the dish immediately.

Nutritional Values (per serving):

Calories: 230 | Fat: 9g | Saturated Fat: 3g | Cholesterol: 80mg | Sodium: 690mg | Carbohydrates: 9g | Fiber: 2g | Sugar: 4g | Protein: 27g

BALSAMIC GLAZED CHICKEN

Ingredients:

- ½ lb boneless, skinless chicken breasts
- ¼ tsp salt
- ¼ tsp black pepper
- 1 tbsp olive oil
- ¼ cup balsamic vinegar
- ½ tbsp honey
- ½ tbsp Dijon mustard
- ½ tsp minced garlic
- ¼ tsp dried rosemary

Instructions:

1. Add salt and black pepper to the chicken breasts.
2. Heat up the olive oil in a non-stick pan over medium heat.
3. Add the chicken breasts and cook for 5–6 minutes per side or until they are fully cooked and browned.

4. Mix the balsamic vinegar, honey, Dijon mustard, minced garlic, and dried rosemary in a small bowl with a whisk.
5. Pour the glaze made from balsamic vinegar over the chicken breasts in the pan. Cook the chicken for 2-3 minutes on low heat until the glaze thickens and evenly coats the chicken.
6. Remove the chicken from the pan before cutting it into desired pieces.
7. Divide the chicken with balsamic glaze between two plates and serve with any side dishes you like.

Nutritional Values (per serving):

Calories: 270 | Fat: 10g | Saturated Fat: 2g | Cholesterol: 80mg | Sodium: 560mg | Carbohydrates: 14g | Fiber: 0g | Sugar: 12g | Protein: 30g

SAUSAGE, PEPPERS, AND ONIONS SKILLETS

Ingredients:

- ½ lb Italian turkey sausage, sliced
- 1 tbsp olive oil
- 1 cup sliced bell peppers (any color)
- 1 cup sliced onion
- ¼ cup low-sodium chicken broth
- ¼ cup low-sodium marinara sauce
- ¼ tsp dried oregano
- ¼ tsp dried basil

Instructions:

1. In a big nonstick skillet, warm the olive oil over medium heat. Add the sliced turkey sausage to the pan and cook for 4-5 minutes, turning the slices occasionally until they are browned on all sides. From the skillet, take out the sausage, and set it aside.
2. In the same pan, combine the bell peppers and onions. Cook the vegetables for 5 to 6 minutes while occasionally stirring until they are soft.

3. Return the cooked sausage to the skillet. Stir in the chicken broth, marinara sauce, dried oregano, and dried basil. Continue cooking the mixture for an additional 3-4 minutes, or until it is heated through and reaches the desired temperature.
4. Divide the sausage, peppers, and onions skillet between two plates and serve.

Nutritional Values (per serving):

Calories: 340 | Fat: 19g | Saturated Fat: 4g | Cholesterol: 70mg | Sodium: 930mg | Carbohydrates: 20g | Fiber: 4g | Sugar: 9g | Protein: 24g

ROSEMARY LEMON PORK CHOPS

Ingredients:

- ½ lb boneless pork chops (about 2 chops)
- ¼ tsp salt
- ¼ tsp black pepper
- 1 tbsp olive oil
- ¼ cup lemon juice
- ¼ cup low-sodium chicken broth
- ½ tsp minced garlic
- ½ tsp dried rosemary

Instructions:

1. Add salt and black pepper to the pork chops.
2. Heat up the olive oil in a non-stick pan over medium heat. Once the pork chops have been added to the pan, cook them for approximately 4-5 minutes on each side.
3. Using a whisk, combine the lemon juice, chicken broth, minced garlic, and dried rosemary in a small bowl until they are well mixed. Pour the mixture over the pork chops in the pan.
4. Keep cooking the sauce on low heat for another three to four minutes or until it starts to get a little thicker.

5. Divide the rosemary lemon pork chops between two plates and serve with your choice of side dishes.

Nutritional Values (per serving):

Calories: 300 | Fat: 18g | Saturated Fat: 4g | Cholesterol: 90mg | Sodium: 430mg | Carbohydrates: 3g | Fiber: 0g | Sugar: 1g | Protein: 29g

MOROCCAN-SPICED BEEF STEW

Ingredients:

- ½ lb lean beef stew meat
- ¼ tsp salt
- ¼ tsp black pepper
- 1 tbsp olive oil
- ½ cup chopped onion
- ½ cup chopped carrot
- ½ cup chopped celery
- ½ cup low-sodium beef broth
- ½ cup canned diced tomatoes, undrained
- ½ tsp ground cumin
- ½ tsp ground coriander
- ¼ tsp ground cinnamon
- ¼ tsp paprika
- ¼ cup chopped fresh cilantro

Instructions:

1. Season the beef stew meat with salt and black pepper.
2. In a large pot or Dutch oven, heat the olive oil over medium heat. Cook, turning the meat regularly, for 4-5 minutes, or until all sides are browned. Remove the steak from the saucepan and place it on a plate or bowl.
3. To the same saucepan, add the onion, carrot, and celery. Cook for 4-5 minutes, stirring periodically, until the vegetables are softened.
4. Add the cooked beef back to the pot. Incorporate the beef broth, diced tomatoes, cumin, coriander, cinnamon, and paprika. Bring the ingredients to a boil.

5. Reduce the heat to low, cover the pot, and let it simmer for an hour to an hour and a half, or until the meat is cooked.

6. Just before serving, add the chopped fresh cilantro to the stew and mix thoroughly to ensure it is equally distributed throughout the dish. Serve the Moroccan-spiced beef stew in separate dishes.

Nutritional Values (per serving):

Calories: 350 | Fat: 16g | Saturated Fat: 4g | Cholesterol: 85mg | Sodium: 540mg | Carbohydrates: 17g | Fiber: 4g | Sugar: 6g | Protein: 34g

SPINACH AND FETA STUFFED CHICKEN BREASTS

Ingredients:

- 2 boneless, skinless chicken breasts
- ¼ tsp salt
- ¼ tsp black pepper
- ½ cup chopped fresh spinach
- ¼ cup crumbled feta cheese
- 1 tbsp olive oil
- ¼ cup low-sodium chicken broth

Instructions:

1. Set the oven's temperature to 375°F (190°C).
2. Carefully cut a horizontal pocket into each chicken breast with a sharp knife without cutting all the way through.
3. Season the chicken breasts to taste with salt and black pepper.
4. Fill each chicken breast pocket with half of the chopped spinach and crumbled feta cheese.
5. Heat the olive oil in a big oven-safe skillet over medium heat until it is hot.
6. Cook the chicken breasts that have been packed with filling for 4 to 5 minutes on each side, or until browned.
7. After adding the chicken broth to the pan, place it in a preheated oven. Bake for 15 to 20 minutes, or until the chicken is completely cooked through.

8. Serve the spinach and feta stuffed chicken breasts with your choice of side dishes on two platters.

Nutritional Values (per serving):

Calories: 300 | Fat: 15g | Saturated Fat: 4g | Cholesterol: 100mg | Sodium: 620mg | Carbohydrates: 2g | Fiber: 1g | Sugar: 1g | Protein: 36g

ASIAN TURKEY LETTUCE WRAPS

Ingredients:

- ½ lb lean ground turkey
- ¼ cup hoisin sauce
- 1 tbsp low-sodium soy sauce
- ½ tbsp rice vinegar
- ½ tbsp grated fresh ginger
- ½ tbsp minced garlic
- ½ cup chopped water chestnuts
- ¼ cup chopped green onions
- ¼ cup chopped fresh cilantro
- 6 large iceberg or butter lettuce
- leaves
- Optional toppings: chopped peanuts, Sriracha sauce

Instructions:

1. Spoon-break ground turkey in a non-stick skillet over medium heat. Cook until browned and fully cooked through.
2. Mix hoisin sauce, soy sauce, rice vinegar, grated ginger, and minced garlic in a small bowl. After the turkey is cooked, pour the sauce over it and stir until the sauce is evenly distributed and fully combined with the turkey.
3. Add the chopped water chestnuts, green onions, and fresh cilantro to the skillet and stir them in until they are well combined with the other ingredients. Cook the combined ingredients for an additional 2-3 minutes until they are heated through and ready to be served.
4. Using a spoon, place the ground turkey mixture into the lettuce leaves. Add

optional toppings such as chopped
peanuts or Sriracha sauce, if desired.

5. Take lettuce leaves and fold them
    around the filling, making sure to wrap
    them securely. Serve immediately.

Nutritional Values (per serving):

Calories: 230 | Fat: 7g | Saturated Fat: 2g |
Cholesterol: 60mg | Sodium: 860mg |
Carbohydrates: 20g | Fiber: 3g | Sugar: 9g |
Protein: 22g

SEAFOODS RECIPE

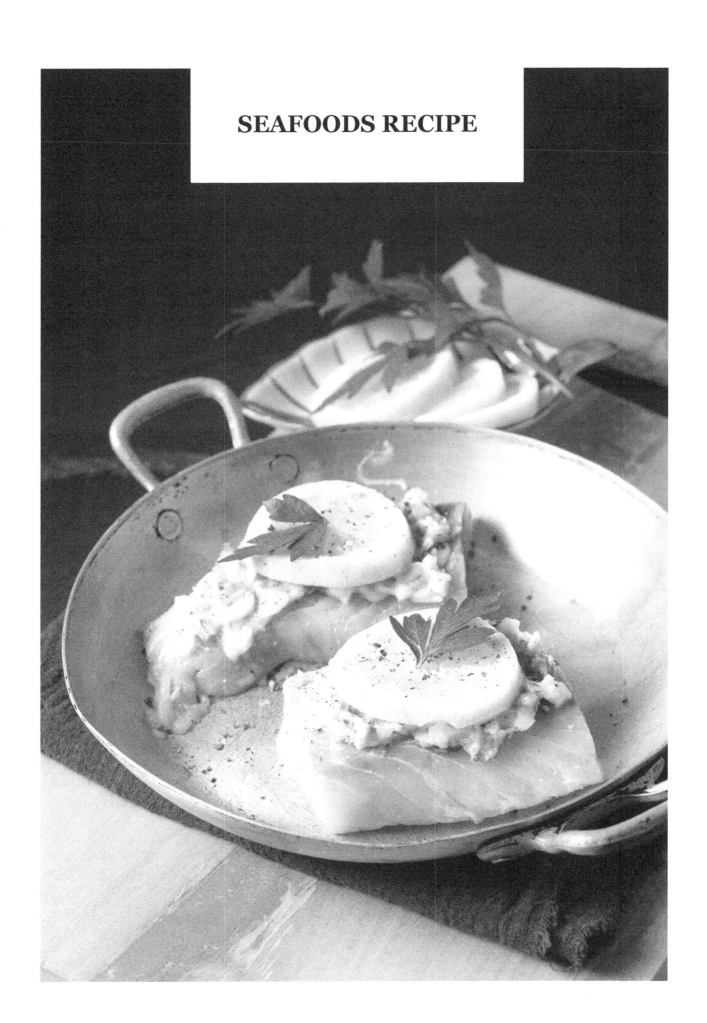

LEMON GARLIC BAKED COD

Ingredients:

- 2 (6 oz) cod fillets
- 2 tbsp olive oil
- 2 cloves garlic, minced
- ½ lemon, juiced
- ¼ tsp salt
- ¼ tsp black pepper
- 1 tbsp chopped fresh parsley

Instructions:

1. Set the oven's temperature to 400°F (200°C). Take a baking sheet and cover it with parchment paper to prevent the food from sticking to the surface of the sheet.
2. Combine olive oil, minced garlic, lemon juice, salt, and black pepper in a small bowl and whisk all the ingredients together until they are fully blended.
3. Put the cod fillets on the baking sheet that has been prepared and brush them with the lemon-garlic mixture.
4. Cook the fish in the oven for a duration of 12 to 15 minutes or until it becomes tender enough to break apart effortlessly using a fork.
5. Garnish with chopped fresh parsley and serve.

Nutritional Values (per serving):

Calories: 210 | Fat: 11g | Saturated Fat: 1.5g | Cholesterol: 65mg | Sodium: 390mg | Carbohydrates: 2g | Fiber: 0g | Sugar: 0g | Protein: 24g

SHRIMP AND VEGGIE STIR-FRY

Ingredients:

- 1 tbsp olive oil
- ½ lb raw shrimp, peeled and deveined
- ½ cup sliced bell pepper
- ½ cup sliced onion
- ½ cup snow peas
- ½ cup broccoli florets
- 1 tbsp low-sodium soy sauce
- 1 tbsp oyster sauce
- ½ tbsp honey
- ½ tbsp cornstarch
- ¼ cup water

Instructions:

1. Begin by heating the olive oil in a large frying pan or wok over medium-high heat.
2. Once the oil reaches the required temperature, add the shrimp to the frying pan and cook for 2-3 minutes on each side, or until it turns a nice pink color and is thoroughly cooked. Remove the shrimp from the skillet and set it aside for later use.
3. In the same skillet, combine the bell pepper, onion, snow peas, and broccoli. Cook for 4-5 minutes, stirring periodically, until the vegetables are soft and cooked to your satisfaction.
4. In a small mixing bowl, combine soy sauce, oyster sauce, honey, cornstarch, and water until well combined.
5. Return the cooked shrimp to the pan and stir until the sauce is uniformly spread and all of the ingredients are properly mixed. Cook for another 2-3 minutes, or until the sauce has thickened to the desired consistency. Stir occasionally to prevent the sauce from burning or sticking to the pan.
6. Serve the shrimp and vegetable stir-fry on two dishes.

Nutritional Values (per serving):

Calories: 280 | Fat: 10g | Saturated Fat: 1.5g | Cholesterol: 170mg | Sodium: 840mg | Carbohydrates: 21g | Fiber: 3g | Sugar: 9g | Protein: 26g

PAN-SEARED SCALLOPS WITH GARLIC SPINACH

Ingredients:

- 6 large sea scallops, patted dry
- 1 tbsp olive oil
- 1 tbsp unsalted butter
- 1 clove garlic, minced
- 4 cups fresh spinach

- ¼ tsp salt
- ¼ tsp black pepper
- ¼ tsp crushed red pepper flakes (optional)

Instructions:

1. In a large pan, heat a half tablespoon of olive oil over medium-high heat.
2. Season the scallops with salt and black pepper to taste. Place the scallops in the heated pan and cook for approximately 2-3 minutes on both sides until they are evenly cooked and achieve a golden-brown color. Once done, transfer the scallops from the pan onto a plate.
3. Using the same pan, heat the remaining half tablespoon of olive oil and the butter until the butter is fully melted and the oil is hot. Place the diced garlic into the pan and sauté for about a minute or until a pleasant aroma emanates from the garlic.
4. Add fresh spinach, salt, black pepper, and crushed red pepper flakes (if using) to the pan and stir everything together until the spinach wilts and becomes tender.
5. Divide the garlic spinach evenly between two plates, place the cooked scallops on top of the spinach, and serve immediately.

Nutritional Values (per serving):

Calories: 260 | Fat: 17g | Saturated Fat: 5g | Cholesterol: 45mg | Sodium: 700mg | Carbohydrates: 6g | Fiber: 2g | Sugar: 1g | Protein: 20g

SALMON WITH DILL YOGURT SAUCE

Ingredients:

- 2 (4 oz) salmon fillets
- ½ tsp salt
- ¼ tsp black pepper
- ½ cup plain Greek yogurt
- 1 tbsp chopped fresh dill
- 1 tsp lemon juice
- ½ tsp garlic powder

Instructions:

1. Set the oven to 425°F (220°C) and turn it on. Put parchment paper on a baking sheet.
2. Add salt and black pepper to the salmon filets. Arrange them on the baking sheet with the skin side facing down.
3. Allow the salmon to bake for a duration of 12-15 minutes or until it is thoroughly cooked and can be effortlessly flaked apart using a fork.
4. In a small bowl, mix together fresh dill, garlic powder, lemon juice, and Greek yogurt until the ingredients are well combined.
5. Serve the cooked salmon with a dollop of dill yogurt sauce.

Nutritional Values (per serving):

Calories: 300 | Fat: 15g | Saturated Fat: 3g | Cholesterol: 80mg | Sodium: 720mg | Carbohydrates: 3g | Fiber: 0g | Sugar: 2g | Protein: 35g

CRAB CAKES WITH LEMON AIOLI

Ingredients:

For the crab cakes:

- 8 oz lump crabmeat, drained
- ¼ cup whole wheat breadcrumbs
- ¼ cup chopped fresh parsley
- ¼ cup chopped green onions
- ¼ cup mayonnaise
- ¼ tsp salt
- ¼ tsp black pepper
- 1 large egg, lightly beaten
- 2 tbsp olive oil

For the lemon aioli:

- ¼ cup mayonnaise
- 1 tbsp lemon juice
- 1 tsp grated lemon zest
- ¼ tsp garlic powder

Instructions:

1. In a large bowl, combine the crabmeat, breadcrumbs, parsley, green onions, mayonnaise, salt, black pepper, and beaten egg. Gently mix until well combined.
2. Make crab cakes from each of the four equal parts of the mixture.
3. To prepare the crab cakes, it is recommended to heat a nonstick skillet over medium heat and add olive oil to the skillet. After heating the skillet, the crab cakes should be cooked for around 3-4 minutes on each side until they achieve a consistent, golden brown color and are uniformly heated throughout.
4. Combine all the ingredients for the lemon aioli in a small bowl and mix them together thoroughly.
5. Add a dollop of lemon aioli to the crab cakes and serve.

Nutritional Values (per serving):

Calories: 420 | Fat: 32g | Saturated Fat: 4.5g | Cholesterol: 135mg | Sodium: 980mg | Carbohydrates: 10g | Fiber: 1g | Sugar: 2g | Protein: 20g

ONE-PAN SHRIMP AND ASPARAGUS

Ingredients:

- ½ lb raw shrimp, peeled and deveined
- ½ lb asparagus, trimmed
- 1 tbsp olive oil
- ½ lemon, juiced
- 2 cloves garlic, minced
- ¼ tsp salt
- ¼ tsp black pepper
- ¼ tsp crushed red pepper flakes (optional)

Instructions:

1. To start, you should preheat your oven to 400°F (200°C). Following this, prepare your baking sheet by covering it with parchment paper.

2. Combine the prawns, asparagus, olive oil, lemon juice, garlic, salt, black pepper, and optional crushed red pepper flakes (if desired) in a spacious bowl, and mix thoroughly. Spread the shrimp and asparagus mixture evenly on the prepared baking sheet.
3. Cook the shrimp and asparagus for a duration of 10-12 minutes, or until the shrimp have turned pink and are fully cooked while the asparagus has reached a state of tenderness.
4. Divide the one-pan shrimp and asparagus between two plates and serve.

Nutritional Values (per serving):

Calories: 190 | Fat: 8g | Saturated Fat: 1g | Cholesterol: 145mg | Sodium: 720mg | Carbohydrates: 9g | Fiber: 3g | Sugar: 3g | Protein: 22g

BAKED TILAPIA WITH MEDITERRANEAN SALSA

Ingredients:

- 2 (6 oz) tilapia fillets
- ½ cup chopped tomatoes
- ¼ cup chopped cucumber
- ¼ cup chopped red onion
- ¼ cup chopped Kalamata olives
- ¼ cup chopped fresh parsley
- 1 tbsp olive oil
- ½ lemon, juiced
- ¼ tsp salt
- ¼ tsp black pepper

Instructions:

1. To start, you should preheat your oven to 400°F (200°C). Following this, prepare your baking sheet by covering it with parchment paper.
2. Season the tilapia fillets with salt and black pepper to taste. Then place them on the prepared baking sheet.
3. Cook the fish in the oven for approximately 12 to 15 minutes or until

it becomes tender enough to be separated easily with a fork.

4. In a medium bowl, mix together the tomatoes, cucumber, red onion, Kalamata olives, parsley, olive oil, and lemon juice until all the ingredients are well combined.
5. Serve the cooked tilapia topped with Mediterranean salsa.

Nutritional Values (per serving):

Calories: 300 | Fat: 13g | Saturated Fat: 2g | Cholesterol: 85mg | Sodium: 700mg | Carbohydrates: 9g | Fiber: 2g | Sugar: 4g | Protein: 36g

EASY CLAM SPAGHETTI

Ingredients:

- 4 oz whole wheat spaghetti
- 1 tbsp olive oil
- ¼ cup chopped onion
- 2 cloves garlic, minced
- 1 (6.5 oz) can of chopped clams, drained (reserve the juice)
- ¼ cup clam juice (from the can)
- ¼ cup chopped fresh parsley
- ¼ tsp crushed red pepper flakes (optional)
- ¼tsp black pepper

Instructions:

1. Cook the whole wheat spaghetti according to package instructions until al dente. Drain the mixture and set it aside.
2. Heat the olive oil in a large skillet over medium heat. Afterward, include the onion and garlic, and let it cook for approximately 3-4 minutes until the onion turns translucent.
3. Introduce the chopped clams, clam juice, parsley, black pepper, and optionally crushed red pepper flakes into the skillet. Cook for 5 minutes, stirring occasionally.
4. Toss the cooked spaghetti with the clam sauce. Divide the spaghetti evenly

between two plates and serve immediately.

Nutritional Values (per serving):

Calories: 350 | Fat: 9g | Saturated Fat: 1g | Cholesterol: 20mg | Sodium: 570mg | Carbohydrates: 50g | Fiber: 6g | Sugar: 2g | Protein: 20g

SEARED AHI TUNA WITH MANGO SALSA

Ingredients:

- 2 (4 oz) ahi tuna steaks
- ½ tsp salt
- ¼ tsp black pepper
- 1 tbsp olive oil

For the mango salsa:

- ½ cup diced mango
- ¼ cup diced red bell pepper
- ¼ cup chopped red onion
- ¼ cup chopped fresh cilantro
- ½ jalapeño, seeded and minced
- ½ lime, juiced
- ¼ tsp salt

Instructions:

1. Pat the ahi tuna steaks dry with paper towels and season them with salt and black pepper.
2. Warm up the olive oil using a non-stick pan on medium to high heat. Add the tuna steaks to the pan and sear them on each side for 1-2 minutes, or until the outer layer is seared and the center is still pink.
3. For the mango salsa, combine freshly diced mango, finely chopped red bell pepper, and red onion in a medium-sized bowl. Add in the minced jalapeño, fresh cilantro, lime juice, and salt. Mix all the ingredients together thoroughly.
4. Serve the seared ahi tuna topped with mango salsa.

Nutritional Values (per serving):

Calories: 270 | Fat: 11g | Saturated Fat: 2g | Cholesterol: 45mg | Sodium: 810mg | Carbohydrates: 13g | Fiber: 2g | Sugar: 10g | Protein: 30g

SEAFOOD PAELLA

Ingredients:

- 1 tbsp olive oil
- ¼ cup chopped onion
- ¼ cup chopped red bell pepper
- ¼ cup chopped green bell pepper
- ½ cup Arborio rice
- 1 cup low-sodium chicken or vegetable broth
- ¼ tsp saffron threads
- ¼ tsp paprika
- ¼ tsp salt
- ¼ tsp black pepper
- ½ cup canned diced tomatoes drained
- ½ cup frozen peas, thawed
- ½ lb mixed seafood (shrimp, scallops, mussels, and/or squid)
- ¼ cup chopped fresh parsley

Instructions:

1. Begin by warming up the olive oil in a generously-sized skillet set to medium heat.
2. Toss in the diced onion, red bell pepper, and green bell pepper, and allow the mixture to cook for around 4 to 5 minutes or until the vegetables have softened to your liking.
3. Add the Arborio rice to the skillet, stirring to coat the rice with oil. Cook for 2 minutes, stirring occasionally.
4. Stir in the chicken or vegetable broth, saffron threads, paprika, salt, black pepper, and diced tomatoes. Bring the combination to a boiling point, then reduce the temperature and allow it to simmer for 15 minutes, stirring occasionally.
5. Add the peas and mixed seafood to the skillet. After covering the dish, allow it to cook for an additional 10-15 minutes until the rice has softened and the seafood has been fully cooked.
6. Lastly, add the chopped fresh parsley and serve.

Nutritional Values (per serving):

Calories: 390 | Fat: 9g | Saturated Fat: 1.5g | Cholesterol: 120mg | Sodium: 710mg | Carbohydrates: 52g | Fiber: 4g | Sugar: 5g | Protein: 26g

BAKED COD WITH CHERRY TOMATOES AND OLIVES

Ingredients:

- 2 (6 oz) cod fillets
- ½ cup cherry tomatoes, halved
- ¼ cup pitted Kalamata olives, halved
- 1 tbsp olive oil
- ½ lemon, juiced
- ¼ tsp salt
- ¼ tsp black pepper
- ¼ cup chopped fresh basil

Instructions:

1. Warm up the oven to a temperature of 400°F (200°C). Put parchment paper on a baking sheet.
2. Prepare the baking sheet in advance and arrange the cod fillets on it. To enhance their flavor, sprinkle a pinch of black pepper and salt over them
3. Combine the cherry tomatoes, Kalamata olives, olive oil, and lemon juice in a medium bowl. Mix well.
4. Distribute the mixture of tomatoes and olives on top of the cod fillets.
5. Put the prepared dish inside the oven and cook for roughly 12 to 15 minutes or until the fish can be easily separated with a fork.
6. Garnish with chopped fresh basil and serve.

Nutritional Values (per serving):

Calories: 240 | Fat: 10g | Saturated Fat: 1.5g | Cholesterol: 65mg | Sodium: 670mg | Carbohydrates: 6g | Fiber: 1g | Sugar: 3g | Protein: 30g

GARLIC BUTTER SCALLOPS

Ingredients:

- 8 large sea scallops, patted dry
- 1 tbsp olive oil
- 2 tbsp unsalted butter
- 2 cloves garlic, minced
- ¼ tsp salt
- ¼ tsp black pepper
- ¼ cup chopped fresh parsley
- ½ lemon, juiced

Instructions:

1. Heat the olive oil in a large nonstick skillet over medium heat.
2. When the oil is hot enough, carefully add the scallops to the pan and cook for 2 to 3 minutes on each side, or until well cooked and a crisp golden brown. Place the scallops on a platter after removing them from the pan.
3. Melt the butter in a pan over medium heat until thoroughly melted.
4. Once the butter has melted, add the garlic and sauté for 1 to 2 minutes, or until the perfume of the garlic can be detected.
5. Add the scallops back to the skillet with the melted butter and season with salt and black pepper to taste. Cook for another 1-2 minutes, or until the scallops are heated through and fully cooked. Continue to gently stir them until they are evenly cooked on both sides.
6. Once the scallops have done cooking, stir with the chopped parsley and lemon juice until well combined. On two plates, serve the scallops with garlic butter.

Nutritional Values (per serving):

Calories: 240 | Fat: 16g | Saturated Fat: 6g | Cholesterol: 65mg| Sodium: 540mg | Carbohydrates: 6g | Fiber: 0g | Sugar: 0g | Protein: 20g

LEMON HERB BAKED SALMON

Ingredients:

- 2 (6 oz) salmon fillets
- 1 tbsp olive oil
- ½ lemon, juiced
- ¼ tsp salt
- ¼ tsp black pepper
- ¼ tsp dried thyme
- ¼ tsp dried rosemary
- ¼ tsp dried oregano
- ½ lemon, sliced

Instructions:

1. To begin, preheat your oven to 375°F (190°C) and then prepare a baking sheet by lining it with parchment paper. This will prevent the food from sticking to the sheet during the cooking process.
2. Arrange the salmon fillets onto the prepared baking sheet, making sure to leave some space between each fillet. This will ensure that they cook evenly and thoroughly. Sprinkle with salt, black pepper, thyme, rosemary, and oregano, and then drizzle with olive oil and lemon juice.
3. Place the lemon slices on top of the salmon fillets.
4. Cook the salmon in the oven for a duration of 12 to 15 minutes or until it reaches a point where it can be easily separated with a fork.
5. Divide the lemon herb baked salmon between two plates and serve.

Nutritional Values (per serving):

Calories: 300 | Fat: 18g | Saturated Fat: 3g | Cholesterol: 85mg | Sodium: 370mg | Carbohydrates: 2g | Fiber: 1g | Sugar: 0g | Protein: 31g

SPICY CAJUN SHRIMP SKILLET

Ingredients:

- 1 tbsp olive oil
- ½ lb shrimp, peeled and deveined
- ¼ cup chopped onion
- ¼ cup chopped bell pepper
- ¼ cup chopped celery
- ¼ cup low-sodium vegetable broth
- ¼ cup canned diced tomatoes
- ¼ tsp cajun seasoning
- ¼ tsp salt
- ¼ tsp black pepper
- ¼ cup chopped green onions

Instructions:

1. To begin the cooking process, heat the olive oil in a large skillet or wok over medium-high heat.
2. Once the oil is hot, add the shrimp and cook for about 2-3 minutes on both sides, or until it is a lovely shade of pink and well cooked. Remove the shrimp from the skillet and set it aside for later use.
3. Add the onion, bell pepper, and celery to the same skillet. Cook the vegetables for 4-5 minutes, or until they reach the desired consistency.
4. Combine the vegetable broth, diced tomatoes, Cajun seasoning, salt, and black pepper in a mixing bowl. Heat the mixture over low-medium heat for about 5-6 minutes, stirring regularly, until the sauce thickens somewhat. Return the shrimp to the skillet and cook for a further 1-2 minutes, or until they are completely heated through.
5. Stir in the green onions, if using. Serve the spicy Cajun shrimp skillet between two dishes.

Nutritional Values (per serving):

Calories: 230 | Fat: 9g | Saturated Fat: 1.5g | Cholesterol: 180mg | Sodium: 630mg | Carbohydrates: 9g | Fiber: 2g | Sugar: 4g | Protein: 29g

MISO-GLAZED SALMON

Ingredients:

- 2 (6 oz) salmon fillets
- 1 tbsp white miso paste
- 1 tbsp mirin
- 1 tbsp low-sodium soy sauce

- ½ tsp sesame oil
- ½ tsp honey
- ½ tsp grated ginger

Instructions:

1. Warm up the oven to a temperature of 400°F (200°C). Put parchment paper on a baking sheet.
2. Whisk the miso paste, mirin, soy sauce, sesame oil, honey, and grated ginger together in a small bowl.
3. Lay the salmon fillets on the prepared baking sheet and brush them with the miso mixture.
4. Arrange the salmon on a baking sheet and place it in the oven, baking for approximately 10-12 minutes or until it becomes flaky and can be easily separated with a fork.
5. Divide the miso-glazed salmon evenly between two plates and serve immediately.

Nutritional Values (per serving):

Calories: 280 | Fat: 11g | Saturated Fat: 2g | Cholesterol: 85mg | Sodium: 510mg | Carbohydrates: 7g | Fiber: 0g | Sugar: 4g | Protein: 37g

SHRIMP SCAMPI

Ingredients:

- 1 tbsp olive oil
- ½ lb shrimp, peeled and deveined
- 2 cloves garlic, minced
- ¼ cup dry white wine
- ¼ cup low-sodium chicken broth
- 1 tbsp lemon juice
- ¼ tsp red pepper flakes
- ¼ tsp salt
- ¼ tsp black pepper
- ¼ cup chopped fresh parsley

Instructions:

1. Using a large non-stick skillet, heat up the olive oil over a medium-high heat setting.

2. Place the shrimp into the pan and allow it to cook for approximately 2-3 minutes on each side until it turns pink in color and is fully cooked. Remove the shrimp from the frying pan and transfer them to a dish using a slotted spoon.

3. In the same skillet, add the garlic and cook it for about 1 minute or until it becomes fragrant.

4. In a saucepan, combine chicken broth, white wine, lemon juice, red pepper flakes, salt, and black pepper. Mix the ingredients thoroughly until the mixture starts to simmer.

5. Let the mixture cook for 3-4 minutes or until the sauce has reduced slightly to your desired consistency.

6. Once the sauce has reduced slightly, add the prawns back to the frying pan and continue cooking for another 1-2 minutes or until they are fully warmed through.

7. Stir in the chopped fresh parsley. Divide the shrimp scampi between two plates and serve.

Nutritional Values (per serving):

Calories: 210 | Fat: 9g | Saturated Fat: 1.5g | Cholesterol: 180mg | Sodium: 740mg | Carbohydrates: 3g | Fiber: 0g | Sugar: 1g | Protein: 29g

LEMON GARLIC BAKED TILAPIA

Ingredients:

- 2 (6 oz) tilapia fillets
- 1 tbsp olive oil
- 2 cloves garlic, minced
- ½ lemon, juiced
- ¼ tsp salt
- ¼ tsp black pepper
- ¼ tsp paprika
- ¼ cup chopped fresh parsley

Instructions:

1. Warm up the oven to a temperature of 400°F (200°C).

2. Cover a baking sheet with parchment paper, and then place the tilapia fillets on the baking sheet.

3. Combine minced garlic, lemon juice, olive oil, salt, black pepper, and paprika in a small bowl and mix all the ingredients together thoroughly. Blend well.

4. Spread the garlic sauce over the fillets of tilapia.

5. Cook the fish in the oven for a duration of 12 to 15 minutes or until it becomes tender enough to break apart effortlessly using a fork.

6. Garnish with chopped fresh parsley and serve.

Nutritional Values (per serving):

Calories: 230 | Fat: 10g | Saturated Fat: 1.5g | Cholesterol: 85mg | Sodium: 420mg | Carbohydrates: 3g | Fiber: 1g | Sugar: 0g | Protein: 34g

SHRIMP AND SPINACH STUFFED PORTOBELLO MUSHROOMS

Ingredients:

- 2 large Portobello mushroom caps, stems removed
- 1 tbsp olive oil
- ½ lb shrimp, peeled and deveined
- 2 cups baby spinach, chopped
- ¼ cup low-fat cream cheese
- ¼ cup grated Parmesan cheese
- ¼ tsp garlic powder
- ¼ tsp salt
- ¼ tsp black pepper

Instructions:

1. Warm up the oven to a temperature of 400°F (200°C). Line a baking sheet with parchment paper.
2. Place the Portobello mushroom caps, gill-side up, on the prepared baking sheet.
3. Heat the olive oil in a nonstick skillet over medium heat until it is hot. Add the shrimp to

the skillet and cook for 2-3 minutes on each side, or until they are pink and cooked through. Before removing the shrimp from the flame, make sure they have turned a light pink hue to signal they are fully cooked. Take the prawns out of the pan and cut them into small pieces.

4. Cook the chopped spinach in the same skillet for 1-2 minutes, or until it wilts and turns soft.

5. Combine the cooked shrimp, wilted spinach, cream cheese, Parmesan cheese, garlic powder, salt, and black pepper in a medium mixing bowl.

6. Fill the Portobello mushroom caps with the shrimp and spinach mixture.

7. Bake for 12-15 minutes, or until the mushrooms are soft and the cheese has melted.

8. Arrange the stuffed Portobello mushrooms on two dishes and serve immediately.

Nutritional Values (per serving):

Calories: 340 | Fat: 17g | Saturated Fat: 6g | Cholesterol: 180mg | Sodium: 800mg | Carbohydrates: 12g | Fiber: 2g | Sugar: 5g | Protein: 37g

TERIYAKI GLAZED SALMOND

Ingredients:

- 2 (6 oz) salmon fillets
- ¼ cup low-sodium soy sauce
- ¼ cup mirin
- ¼ cup honey
- ½ tsp grated ginger
- ½ tsp minced garlic

Instructions:

1. Before baking, it is recommended to warm up the oven to a temperature of 400°F (200°C). Put parchment paper on a baking sheet.

2. Combine the soy sauce, mirin, honey, ginger, and garlic in a small saucepan. Heat the mixture over medium heat until it simmers, then continue cooking for 5 to 7 minutes until the sauce reaches a slightly thicker consistency.

3. Brush the teriyaki sauce on the salmon fillets and put them on the baking sheet.

4. Put the salmon into the oven and cook it for around 10-12 minutes or until it becomes flaky and separates easily when poked with a fork. Brush with additional teriyaki sauce halfway through the cooking time.

5. Take out the cooked salmon from the oven and use a brush to apply the teriyaki sauce that is left over.

6. Divide the salmon evenly between two plates and serve immediately.

Nutritional Values (per serving):

Calories: 390 | Fat: 11g | Saturated Fat: 2g | Cholesterol: 95mg | Sodium: 720mg | Carbohydrates: 33g | Fiber: 0g | Sugar: 30g | Protein: 35g

SEAFOOD-STUFFED BELL PEPPERS

Ingredients:

- 2 large bell peppers, halved lengthwise and seeded
- ½ lb mixed seafood (shrimp, crab, scallops), cooked and chopped
- ½ cup cooked brown rice
- ¼ cup chopped onion
- ¼ cup chopped tomato
- ¼ cup chopped fresh parsley
- ¼ cup low-fat feta cheese, crumbled
- ¼ tsp salt
- ¼ tsp black pepper

Instructions:

1. Set the oven to 375°F (190°C). Line a baking sheet with parchment paper.

2. Place the bell pepper halves on the prepared baking sheet, cut side up.

3. Mix the cooked seafood, brown rice, onion, tomato, parsley, feta cheese, salt, and black pepper in a medium bowl.

4. Spoon the seafood mixture into the bell pepper halves, pressing down gently to pack the mixture in.

5. Roast the stuffed bell peppers in the oven for around 25-30 minutes or until

the peppers are tender and the filling is heated completely.

6. Divide the stuffed bell peppers evenly between two plates and serve immediately.

Nutritional Values (per serving):

Calories: 290 | Fat: 5g | Saturated Fat: 2g | Cholesterol: 150mg | Sodium: 640mg | Carbohydrates: 29g | Fiber: 5g | Sugar: 8g | Protein: 30g

LEMON GARLIC SHRIMP AND ASPARAGUS

Ingredients:

- ½ lb shrimp, peeled and deveined
- ½ lb asparagus, trimmed
- 2 tbsp olive oil
- 2 cloves garlic, minced
- ½ lemon, juiced
- ¼ tsp salt
- ¼ tsp black pepper

Instructions:

1. Warm up some olive oil in a large nonstick skillet over medium heat. Continue by adding the minced garlic and stirring frequently for a minute.

2. Next, add the shrimp to the skillet and cook for 2 to 3 minutes on each side, or until it turns a delicate pink and is cooked all the way through. When the shrimp is done, remove it from the skillet and set it aside.

3. Add the asparagus to the same skillet and cook for 4 to 5 minutes, or until it is cooked but still has some of its crispness. When the asparagus is done, return the shrimp and season with lemon juice, salt, and black pepper.

4. Toss everything together and cook for another 1 to 2 minutes, or until all of the flavors have melted together and everything is equally heated.

Arrange the shrimp and asparagus on two dishes and serve immediately.

Nutritional Values (per serving):

Calories: 270 | Fat: 15g | Saturated Fat: 2g | Cholesterol: 180mg | Sodium: 590mg |

Carbohydrates: 8g | Fiber: 3g | Sugar: 3g | Protein: 27g

PESTO BAKED SCALLOPS

Ingredients:

- ½ lb large scallops
- ¼ cup prepared basil pesto
- ¼ cup panko breadcrumbs
- ¼ cup grated Parmesan cheese
- 1 tbsp olive oil

Instructions:

1. To start, you should preheat your oven to 400°F (200°C). Following this, prepare your baking sheet by covering it with parchment paper.

2. Prepare the baking dish and arrange the scallops in a way that they are not overlapping, forming a single layer.

3. Spread a thin layer of basil pesto over each scallop using a spoon or brush.

4. Mix the panko breadcrumbs, Parmesan cheese, and olive oil in a small bowl. Sprinkle the breadcrumb mixture evenly over the scallops to create a crispy and flavorful crust.

5. Bake the scallops in the oven for 12-15 minutes or until they are cooked through and the breadcrumb topping is golden brown.

6. Divide the baked scallops evenly between two plates and serve immediately.

Nutritional Values (per serving):

Calories: 330 | Fat: 19g | Saturated Fat: 4g | Cholesterol: 55mg | Sodium: 700mg | Carbohydrates: 13g | Fiber: 1g | Sugar: 1g | Protein: 25g

TILAPIA WITH LEMON CAPER SAUCE

Ingredients:

- 2 (6 oz) tilapia fillets
- 1 tbsp olive oil
- ¼ cup low-sodium chicken broth

- ¼ cup lemon juice
- 2 tbsp capers, drained
- ¼ tsp salt
- ¼ tsp black pepper

Instructions:

1. Start by heating up some olive oil in a non-stick pan over medium-high heat. Place the tilapia fillets gently into the frying pan and cook them until they are crispy and golden brown on each side, which should take around 3 to 4 minutes. Be sure to cook the ingredients thoroughly until they are fully cooked to ensure they are safe to eat.
2. The tilapia should be put on a plate and covered with aluminum foil to keep it warm.
3. Add the chicken broth, lemon juice, capers, salt, and black pepper in the same skillet. Bring the mixture to a simmer and cook it for 2-3 minutes or until the sauce has reduced slightly to your desired consistency.
4. Spoon the lemon caper sauce over the cooked tilapia fillets.
5. Divide the tilapia fillets evenly between two plates and serve immediately.

Nutritional Values (per serving):

Calories: 230 | Fat: 10g | Saturated Fat: 1.5g | Cholesterol: 85mg | Sodium: 540mg | Carbohydrates: 3g | Fiber: 0g | Sugar: 1g | Protein: 34g

SPICY ORANGE GLAZED SHRIMP

Ingredients:

- ½ lb shrimp, peeled and deveined
- ¼ cup fresh orange juice
- 1 tbsp low-sodium soy sauce
- 1 tbsp honey
- ¼ tsp red pepper flakes
- 1 tbsp olive oil
- ¼ tsp salt
- ¼ tsp black pepper

Instructions:

1. Mix the soy sauce, orange juice, honey, and crushed red pepper in a small bowl. Keep it aside.
2. Heat up the olive oil in a non-stick skillet over medium-high heat.
3. To prepare the shrimp, add a pinch of salt and a sprinkle of black pepper, then cook each side for approximately 2-3 minutes until they turn a pink color and are fully cooked.
4. Add the orange sauce to the skillet containing shrimp, and cook for an additional 1-2 minutes until the sauce thickens a bit and completely covers the shrimp.
5. Divide the cooked shrimp evenly between two plates and serve immediately.

Nutritional Values (per serving):

Calories: 240 | Fat: 9g | Saturated Fat: 1.5g | Cholesterol: 180mg | Sodium: 660mg | Carbohydrates: 13g | Fiber: 0g | Sugar: 11g | Protein: 27g

POACHED COD WITH TOMATO SALSA

Ingredients:

- 2 (6 oz) cod fillets
- 1 cup low-sodium vegetable broth
- 1 cup chopped tomatoes
- ¼ cup chopped red onion
- ¼ cup chopped fresh cilantro
- 1 tbsp lime juice
- ¼ tsp salt
- ¼ tsp black pepper

Instructions:

1. Bring the vegetable broth to a simmer over medium heat in a medium saucepan. Carefully place the cod fillets into the saucepan, making sure that they are completely submerged in the broth. Simmer the fish for 5-7 minutes or until it flakes easily with a fork. Once done,

remove the cod from the broth and set it aside on a separate plate.

2. Mix the chopped tomatoes, red onion, cilantro, lime juice, salt, and black pepper in a medium bowl to create the salsa.
3. Divide the poached cod fillets evenly between two plates, and top each fillet with a generous spoonful of tomato salsa.
4. Serve immediately.

Nutritional Values (per serving):

Calories: 170 | Fat: 1g | Saturated Fat: 0g | Cholesterol: 60mg | Sodium: 540mg | Carbohydrates: 9g | Fiber: 2g | Sugar: 5g | Protein: 30g

LOBSTER AND CORN CHOWDER

Ingredients:

- ½ lb cooked lobster meat, chopped
- 1 tbsp olive oil
- ¼ cup chopped onion
- ¼ cup chopped celery
- ¼ cup chopped red bell pepper
- ¼ cup all-purpose flour
- 2 cups low-sodium chicken broth
- 1 cup frozen corn kernels
- 1 cup of low-fat milk
- ¼ tsp salt
- ¼ tsp black pepper

Instructions:

1. Heat the olive oil in a large saucepan over medium heat until it reaches a high temperature. Cook the onion, celery, and red bell pepper in the skillet for 4-5 minutes, turning periodically, until softened.
2. Stir in the flour and heat for 1-2 minutes, or until the flour turns light brown. Pour in the chicken broth gradually, then add the corn, milk, salt, and black pepper, stirring constantly.
3. Once the mixture has reached boiling point, reduce the heat to a gentle simmer. Stir the ingredients occasionally while cooking, which should take around 10-12 minutes, or until the chowder reaches the appropriate thickness.

4. Stir in the cooked lobster meat and simmer for an additional 2-3 minutes, or until the lobster meat is well heated.
5. Divide the chowder between two dishes and serve right away.

Nutritional Values (per serving):

Calories: 420 | Fat: 12g | Saturated Fat: 2g | Cholesterol: 135mg | Sodium: 790mg | Carbohydrates: 47g | Fiber: 5g | Sugar: 12g | Protein: 34g

SOUPS RECIPES

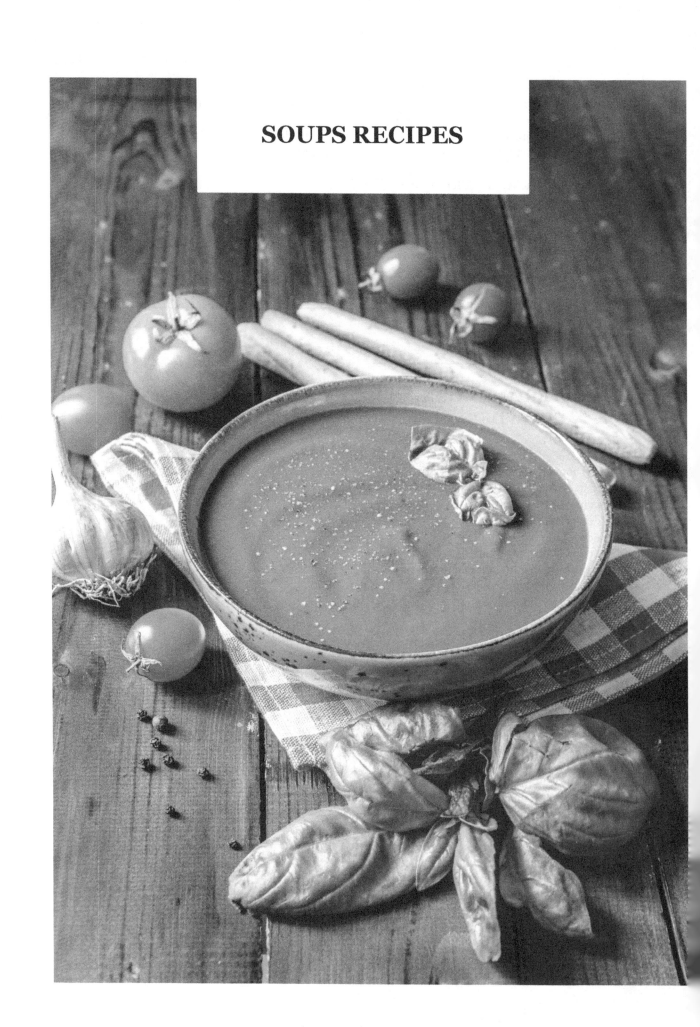

TOMATO BASIL SOUP

Ingredients:

- 1 tbsp olive oil
- ½ cup chopped onion
- 2 cloves garlic, minced
- 2 cups canned crushed tomatoes, no salt added
- 1 cup low-sodium vegetable broth
- ¼ cup chopped fresh basil
- ¼ tsp black pepper
- ¼ tsp salt

Instructions:

1. Heat up some olive oil in a medium-sized saucepan over medium heat. After the oil is heated, add the minced garlic and chopped onion to the pan, and cook them until they become soft and tender, which should take around 4 to 5 minutes.
2. Add the crushed tomatoes, vegetable broth, chopped basil, black pepper, and salt to the mixture and stir until all the ingredients are well combined.
3. The combination is heated until it reaches boiling point, then the heat is reduced, and the mixture is allowed to simmer for 30 minutes.
4. If you prefer a smoother soup, use an immersion blender to puree the mixture until it reaches your desired consistency.
5. After dividing the soup evenly into two bowls, it is now ready to be served.

Nutritional Values (per serving):

Calories: 160 | Fat: 7g | Saturated Fat: 1g | Cholesterol: 0mg | Sodium: 480mg | Carbohydrates: 23g | Fiber: 6g | Sugar: 13g | Protein: 5g

SPINACH AND WHITE BEAN SOUP

Ingredients:

- 1 tbsp olive oil
- ½ cup chopped onion
- 2 cloves garlic, minced
- 2 cups low-sodium vegetable broth
- 1 (15 oz) can cannellini beans, drained and rinsed
- ½ tsp dried thyme
- ¼ tsp salt
- ¼ tsp black pepper
- 2 cups packed fresh spinach

Instructions:

1. Heat up some olive oil in a medium-sized saucepan over medium heat. After the oil is heated, add the minced garlic and chopped onion to the pan, and cook them until they become soft and tender, which should take around 4 to 5 minutes.
2. Stir in the vegetable broth, cannellini beans, dried thyme, salt, and black pepper.
3. The mixture should be heated until it reaches boiling point, then cooled and simmered for ten minutes.
4. Add the spinach to the soup and cook for an additional 2-3 minutes or until the spinach has wilted. Stir the soup occasionally during this time.
5. After dividing the soup evenly into two bowls, it is now ready to be served.

Nutritional Values (per serving):

Calories: 240 | Fat: 7g | Saturated Fat: 1g | Cholesterol: 0mg | Sodium: 490mg | Carbohydrates: 36g | Fiber: 8g | Sugar: 4g | Protein: 12g

SPICED LENTIL SOUP

Ingredients:

- 1 tbsp olive oil
- ½ cup chopped onion
- ½ cup chopped carrots
- ½ cup chopped celery
- ½ cup dried green lentils, rinsed
- 2 cups low-sodium vegetable broth
- ½ tsp ground cumin
- ¼ tsp ground turmeric
- ¼ tsp paprika

- ¼ tsp salt
- ¼ tsp black pepper

Instructions:

1. Place a medium pot over medium heat and warm the olive oil until it's heated through. Add the chopped onion, carrots, and celery to the pot and cook for 4-5 minutes, stirring occasionally, until the vegetables have softened.
2. Stir in the lentils, vegetable broth, cumin, turmeric, paprika, salt, and black pepper.
3. Apply heat to the mixture until it comes to a boil, then decrease the temperature and let it simmer for around 25-30 minutes until the lentils are tender.
4. After dividing the soup evenly into two bowls, it is now ready to be served.

Nutritional Values (per serving):

Calories: 280 | Fat: 7g | Saturated Fat: 1g | Cholesterol: 0mg | Sodium: 480mg | Carbohydrates: 41g | Fiber: 16g | Sugar: 6g | Protein: 16g

MUSHROOM BARLEY SOUP

Ingredients:

- 1 tbsp olive oil
- ½ cup chopped onion
- ½ cup chopped celery
- ½ cup chopped carrots
- ½ lb fresh mushrooms, sliced
- ¼ cup pearl barley rinsed
- 3 cups low-sodium vegetable broth
- ¼ tsp dried thyme
- ¼ tsp salt
- ¼ tsp black pepper

Instructions:

1. Heat the olive oil in a medium pot over medium heat until it is thoroughly hot. In a pot, sauté the chopped onion, celery, and carrots for 4-5 minutes, stirring regularly, until the veggies have softened.

2. Return the sliced mushrooms to the pot and simmer for 3-4 minutes, stirring periodically, until they have released their liquid and are slightly browned.
3. Add the barley, vegetable broth, thyme, salt, and black pepper to taste.
4. Bring the mixture to a boil before reducing to a low heat and simmering for 40 to 45 minutes, or until the barley is soft and tender.
5. The soup is now ready to be served after being evenly divided into two bowls.

Nutritional Values (per serving):

Calories: 250 | Fat: 7g | Saturated Fat: 1g | Cholesterol: 0mg | Sodium: 480mg | Carbohydrates: 42g | Fiber: 9g | Sugar: 7g | Protein: 9g

BUTTERNUT SQUASH AND APPLE SOUP

Ingredients:

- 1 tbsp olive oil
- ½ cup chopped onion
- ½ cup chopped celery
- ½ cup chopped carrots
- ½ lb butternut squash peeled and cubed
- 1 medium apple, peeled, cored, and chopped
- 2 cups low-sodium vegetable broth
- ¼ tsp ground cinnamon
- ¼ tsp ground nutmeg
- ¼ tsp salt
- ¼ tsp black pepper

Instructions:

1. Place a medium pot over medium heat and warm the olive oil until it's heated through. Add the chopped onion, carrots, and celery to the pot and cook for 4-5 minutes, stirring occasionally, until the vegetables have softened.
2. Add the butternut squash, apple, vegetable broth, cinnamon, nutmeg, salt, and black pepper to the pot and stir until all the ingredients are well combined.
3. Apply heat to the mixture until it comes to a boil, then decrease the temperature

and let it simmer for around 20-25 minutes until the squash is tender.
4. Use an immersion blender to blend the soup until it reaches a smooth and creamy consistency.
5. After dividing the soup evenly into two bowls, it is now ready to be served.

Nutritional Values (per serving):

Calories: 210 | Fat: 7g | Saturated Fat: 1g | Cholesterol: 0mg | Sodium: 480mg | Carbohydrates: 38g | Fiber: 6g | Sugar: 15g | Protein: 3g

CHICKEN AND VEGETABLE SOUP

Ingredients:

- 1 tbsp olive oil
- ½ cup chopped onion
- ½ cup chopped carrots
- ½ cup chopped celery
- 2 cups low-sodium chicken broth
- ½ lb cooked chicken breast, diced
- ½ cup frozen peas
- ¼ tsp dried thyme
- ¼ tsp salt
- ¼ tsp black pepper

Instructions:

1. Place a medium pot over medium heat and warm the olive oil until it's heated through. Add the chopped onion, carrots, and celery to a pot and cook for 4-5 minutes, stirring occasionally, until the vegetables have softened.
2. Add the chicken broth, diced chicken, frozen peas, thyme, salt, and black pepper to the pot and stir until all the ingredients are well combined.
3. Apply heat to the mixture until it comes to a boil, then decrease the temperature and let it simmer for around 15 to 20 minutes or until the veggies are fork-tender.

4. Ladle the soup into two bowls, making sure to portion it evenly, and serve immediately.

Nutritional Values (per serving):

Calories: 290 | Fat: 9g | Saturated Fat: 2g | Cholesterol: 80mg | Sodium: 480mg | Carbohydrates: 18g | Fiber: 4g | Sugar: 5g | Protein: 33g

CREAMY CAULIFLOWER SOUP

Ingredients:

- 1 tbsp olive oil
- ½ cup chopped onion
- ½ cup chopped celery
- ½ cup chopped carrots
- ½ lb cauliflower, chopped
- 2 cups low-sodium vegetable broth
- ¼ cup unsweetened almond milk
- ¼ tsp salt
- ¼ tsp black pepper

Instructions:

1. Heat the olive oil in a medium pot over medium heat until it is thoroughly hot. In a pot, sauté the chopped onion, celery, and carrots for 4-5 minutes, stirring periodically, until the veggies are softened.
2. Combine the cauliflower and vegetable broth in a mixing bowl. When the mixture reaches boiling point, reduce the heat to low, cover the pan, and cook for 15 to 20 minutes, or until the cauliflower is tender.
3. Blend the soup with an immersion blender until it achieves a smooth and creamy consistency.
4. Stir in the almond milk, salt, and black pepper until all of the ingredients are completely blended.
5. The soup is now ready to be served after being evenly divided into two bowls.

Nutritional Values (per serving):

Calories: 160 | Fat: 7g | Saturated Fat: 1g | Cholesterol: 0mg | Sodium: 480mg | Carbohydrates: 22g | Fiber: 6g | Sugar: 8g | Protein: 6g

MINESTRONE SOUP

Ingredients:

- 1 tbsp olive oil
- ½ cup chopped onion
- ½ cup chopped celery
- ½ cup chopped carrots
- ½ cup chopped zucchini
- 2 cups low-sodium vegetable broth
- 1 (15 oz) can dice tomatoes, no salt added
- ½ cup canned kidney beans, drained and rinsed
- ½ cup small pasta (e.g., ditalini)
- ¼ tsp dried basil
- ¼ tsp dried oregano
- ¼ tsp salt
- ¼ tsp black pepper

Instructions:

1. Place a medium pot over medium heat and warm the olive oil until it's heated through.
2. Add the chopped onion, celery, carrots, and zucchini to a pot and cook for 4-5 minutes, stirring occasionally, until the vegetables have softened.
3. Stir in the vegetable broth, diced tomatoes, kidney beans, pasta, basil, oregano, salt, and black pepper.
4. Bring the mixture to a boil, then reduce the heat and let it simmer for around 10-15 minutes or until the pasta is cooked and the vegetables are tender. Stir the soup occasionally during this time.
5. After dividing the soup evenly into two bowls, it is now ready to be served.

Nutritional Values (per serving):

Calories: 320 | Fat: 7g | Saturated Fat: 1g | Cholesterol: 0mg | Sodium: 490mg |

Carbohydrates: 55g | Fiber: 11g | Sugar: 9g | Protein: 14g

POTATO LEEK SOUP

Ingredients:

- 1 tbsp olive oil
- ½ cup chopped leeks (white and light green parts only)
- ½ cup chopped celery
- ½ cup chopped carrots
- ½ lb potatoes, peeled and cubed
- 2 cups low-sodium vegetable broth
- ¼ tsp dried thyme
- ¼ tsp salt
- ¼ tsp black pepper

Instructions:

1. Place a medium pot over medium heat and warm the olive oil until it's heated through. Add the chopped leeks, celery, and carrots to a pot and cook for 4-5 minutes, stirring occasionally, until the vegetables have softened.
2. Stir in the potatoes, vegetable broth, thyme, salt, and black pepper.
3. The mixture should be brought to a boil, then simmered for 20 to 25 minutes or until the potatoes are cooked.
4. Use an immersion blender to blend the soup until it reaches a smooth and creamy consistency.
5. After dividing the soup evenly into two bowls, it is now ready to be served.

Nutritional Values (per serving):

Calories: 220 | Fat: 7g | Saturated Fat: 1g | Cholesterol: 0mg | Sodium: 480mg | Carbohydrates: 37g | Fiber: 5g | Sugar: 5g | Protein: 5g

ROASTED RED PEPPER AND TOMATO SOUP

Ingredients:

- 1 tbsp olive oil

- ½ cup chopped onion
- ½ cup chopped celery
- ½ cup chopped carrots
- ½ lb roasted red peppers chopped
- 2 cups canned crushed tomatoes, no salt added
- 2 cups low-sodium vegetable broth
- ¼ tsp dried basil
- ¼ tsp salt
- ¼ tsp black pepper

Instructions:

1. Place a medium pot over medium heat and warm the olive oil until it's heated through. Add the chopped onion, celery, and carrots, and cook for 4-5 minutes, until softened.
2. Stir in the roasted red peppers, crushed tomatoes, vegetable broth, basil, salt, and black pepper.
3. Apply heat to the mixture until it comes to a boil, then decrease the temperature and let it simmer for around 15 to 20 minutes, or until the veggies are the desired tenderness and can be easily pierced with a fork.
4. Use an immersion blender to blend the soup until it reaches a smooth and creamy consistency.
5. After dividing the soup evenly into two bowls, it is now ready to be served.

Nutritional Values (per serving):

Calories: 190 | Fat: 7g | Saturated Fat: 1g | Cholesterol: 0mg | Sodium: 490mg | Carbohydrates: 30g | Fiber: 7g | Sugar: 13g | Protein: 5g

HEARTY VEGETABLE AND BARLEY SOUP

Ingredients:

- 1 tbsp olive oil
- ½ cup chopped onion
- ½ cup chopped carrots
- ½ cup chopped celery
- ½ cup chopped zucchini
- ½ cup chopped green beans
- ¼ cup pearl barley rinsed
- 3 cups low-sodium vegetable broth
- 1 (15 oz) can dice tomatoes, no salt added
- ¼ tsp dried thyme
- ¼ tsp salt
- ¼ tsp black pepper

Instructions:

1. Place a medium pot over medium heat and warm the olive oil until it's heated through. Add the chopped onion, carrots, celery, zucchini, and green beans to a pot and cook for 4-5 minutes, stirring occasionally, until the vegetables have softened.
2. Stir in the barley, vegetable broth, diced tomatoes, thyme, salt, and black pepper.
3. Apply heat to the mixture until it reaches boiling point, then lower the temperature and let it simmer for around 40 to 45 minutes or until the barley is soft and tender to the touch.
4. After dividing the soup evenly into two bowls, it is now ready to be served.

Nutritional Values (per serving):

Calories: 240 | Fat: 7g | Saturated Fat: 1g | Cholesterol: 0mg | Sodium: 490mg | Carbohydrates: 40g | Fiber: 9g | Sugar: 9g | Protein: 7g

WHITE BEAN AND KALE SOUP

Ingredients:

- 1 tbsp olive oil
- ½ cup chopped onion
- ½ cup chopped carrots
- ½ cup chopped celery
- 2 cups low-sodium vegetable broth
- 1 (15 oz) can cannellini beans, drained and rinsed
- ½ lb kale stemmed and chopped
- ¼ tsp dried rosemary
- ¼ tsp salt
- ¼ tsp black pepper

Instructions:

1. Place a medium pot over medium heat and warm the olive oil until it's heated through. Add the chopped onion, carrots, and celery to a pot and cook for 4-5 minutes, stirring occasionally, until the vegetables have softened.
2. Stir in the vegetable broth, cannellini beans, kale, rosemary, salt, and black pepper.
3. Apply heat to the mixture until it comes to a boil, then decrease the temperature and let it simmer for around 15-20 minutes until the kale is tender.
4. After dividing the soup evenly into two bowls, it is now ready to be served.

Nutritional Values (per serving):

Calories: 290 | Fat: 7g | Saturated Fat: 1g | Cholesterol: 0mg | Sodium: 480mg | Carbohydrates: 45g | Fiber: 11g | Sugar: 5g | Protein: 15g

CREAMY MUSHROOM SOUP

Ingredients:

- 1 tbsp olive oil
- ½ cup chopped onion
- ½ cup chopped celery
- ½ cup chopped carrots
- ½ lb mushrooms, sliced
- 2 cups low-sodium vegetable broth
- ½ cup milk (dairy or non-dairy)
- ¼ tsp dried thyme
- ¼ tsp salt
- ¼ tsp black pepper

Instructions:

1. Place a medium pot over medium heat and warm the olive oil until it's heated through. Add the chopped onion, celery, and carrots, and cook for 4-5 minutes, until softened.
2. Incorporate the mushrooms into the mixture and continue cooking for

another 4-5 minutes until they start to brown and release their juice.
3. Stir in the vegetable broth, milk, thyme, salt, and black pepper.
4. Apply heat to the mixture until it comes to a boil, then decrease the temperature and let it simmer for around 15-20 minutes until the vegetables are tender.
5. After dividing the soup evenly into two bowls, it is now ready to be served.

Nutritional Values (per serving):

Calories: 190 | Fat: 9g | Saturated Fat: 2g | Cholesterol: 5mg | Sodium: 480mg | Carbohydrates: 22g | Fiber: 4g | Sugar: 9g | Protein: 7g

SPICED RED LENTIL SOUP

Ingredients:

- 1 tbsp olive oil
- ½ cup chopped onion
- ½ cup chopped carrots
- ½ cup chopped celery
- ½ cup red lentils, rinsed
- 2 cups low-sodium vegetable broth
- ¼ tsp ground cumin
- ¼ tsp ground turmeric
- ¼ tsp salt
- ¼ tsp black pepper

Instructions:

1. Place a medium pot over medium heat and warm the olive oil until it's heated through. Add the chopped onion, carrots, and celery to a pot and cook for 4-5 minutes, stirring occasionally, until the vegetables have softened.
2. Stir in the red lentils, vegetable broth, cumin, turmeric, salt, and black pepper.
3. Apply heat to the mixture until it comes to a boil, then decrease the temperature and let it simmer for around 20 to 25 minutes or until the lentils are soft.
4. After dividing the soup evenly into two bowls, it is now ready to be served.

Nutritional Values (per serving):

Calories: 260 | Fat: 7g | Saturated Fat: 1g | Cholesterol: 0mg | Sodium: 480mg | Carbohydrates: 37g | Fiber: 15g | Sugar: 4g | Protein: 14g

ZUCCHINI AND CORN CHOWDER

Ingredients:

- 1 tbsp olive oil
- ½ cup chopped onion
- ½ cup chopped zucchini
- ½ cup frozen corn
- 2 cups low-sodium vegetable broth
- ½ cup milk (dairy or non-dairy)
- ¼ tsp dried thyme
- ¼ tsp salt
- ¼ tsp black pepper

Instructions:

1. Place a medium pot over medium heat and warm the olive oil until it's heated through. Add the chopped onion to a pan and cook for 4-5 minutes over medium heat, stirring occasionally, until it has softened.
2. Add the zucchini and corn to the pot and cook for an additional 4-5 minutes, stirring occasionally, until the zucchini has softened.
3. Add the vegetable broth, milk, thyme, salt, and black pepper to the pot and stir until all the ingredients are well combined.
4. Apply heat to the mixture until it comes to a boil, then decrease the temperature and let it simmer for around 10 to 15 minutes to allow the flavors to meld.
5. After dividing the soup evenly into two bowls, it is now ready to be served.

Nutritional Values (per serving):

Calories: 190 | Fat: 9g | Saturated Fat: 2g | Cholesterol: 5mg | Sodium: 480mg |

Carbohydrates: 25g | Fiber: 4g | Sugar: 9g | Protein: 6g

MISO VEGETABLE SOUP

Ingredients:

- 2 cups low-sodium vegetable broth
- ½ cup chopped onion
- ½ cup chopped carrots
- ½ cup chopped zucchini
- ½ cup sliced mushrooms
- ½ cup cubed tofu
- ¼ cup white miso paste
- 2 cups water
- ¼ cup chopped green onions
- ¼ cup chopped fresh cilantro

Instructions:

1. Bring the vegetable broth to a boil in a medium saucepan. Cook the onion, carrots, zucchini, mushrooms, and tofu in a pot for 10-15 minutes, turning regularly, until the vegetables are soft.
2. Whisk together the miso paste and water in a separate bowl until smooth and well blended. Pour the miso mixture into the pot after mixing it together.
3. After whisking together the miso paste and water, simmer the soup for an additional 5 minutes to enable the flavors to blend. Stir occasionally to prevent the bottom of the pot from sticking or scorching.
4. Garnish each bowl of soup with green onions and parsley before serving.

Nutritional Values (per serving):

Calories: 190 | Fat: 5g | Saturated Fat: 1g | Cholesterol: 0mg | Sodium: 510mg | Carbohydrates: 24g | Fiber: 4g | Sugar: 6g | Protein: 12g

CABBAGE AND POTATO SOUP

Ingredients:

- 1 tbsp olive oil
- ½ cup chopped onion
- ½ cup chopped potatoes

- 2 cups shredded cabbage
- 2 cups low-sodium vegetable broth
- ¼ tsp caraway seeds
- ¼ tsp salt
- ¼ tsp black pepper

Instructions:

1. Place a medium pot over medium heat and warm the olive oil until it's heated through. Add the chopped onion and potatoes to a pot and cook for 4-5 minutes over medium heat, stirring occasionally, until the vegetables have softened.
2. Stir in the cabbage, vegetable broth, caraway seeds, salt, and black pepper.
3. Apply heat to the mixture until it comes to a boil, then decrease the temperature and let it simmer for around 15 to 20 minutes or until the cabbage is soft.
4. After dividing the soup evenly into two bowls, it is now ready to be served.

Nutritional Values (per serving):

Calories: 210 | Fat: 7g | Saturated Fat: 1g | Cholesterol: 0mg | Sodium: 480mg | Carbohydrates: 34g | Fiber: 7g | Sugar: 6g | Protein: 5g

PEA AND MINT SOUP

Ingredients:

- 2 cups frozen peas
- 2 cups low-sodium vegetable broth
- ¼ cup chopped fresh mint
- ¼ tsp salt
- ¼ tsp black pepper
- ¼ cup crème fraîche or sour cream (optional)

Instructions:

1. In a medium saucepan, bring the vegetable broth to a boil. Add the frozen peas to the pot and cook for an additional 4-5 minutes, stirring occasionally, until the peas are heated through and tender.
2. Stir in the fresh mint, salt, and black pepper to the pot and stir until all the ingredients are well combined.
3. Use an immersion blender to blend the soup until it reaches a smooth and creamy consistency.
4. Portion the soup into two bowls and add a dollop of crème fraîche or sour cream as a garnish, if desired, before serving.

Nutritional Values (per serving, without crème fraîche):

Calories: 130 | Fat: 1g | Saturated Fat: 0g | Cholesterol: 0mg | Sodium: 490mg | Carbohydrates: 22g | Fiber: 8g | Sugar: 8g | Protein: 8g

POTATO AND LEEK SOUP

Ingredients:

- 1 tbsp olive oil
- ½ cup chopped leeks, white and light green parts only
- ½ cup chopped potatoes
- 2 cups low-sodium vegetable broth
- ¼ tsp dried thyme
- ¼ tsp salt
- ¼ tsp black pepper

Instructions:

1. Place a medium pot over medium heat and warm the olive oil until it's heated through. Add the chopped leeks to the pot and cook for another 4 to 5 minutes, stirring occasionally, until the leeks are soft.
2. Mix in the potatoes, veggie broth, thyme, salt, and black pepper.
3. Apply heat to the mixture until it comes to a boil, then decrease the temperature and let it simmer for around 15 to 20 minutes or until the potatoes become tender.
4. After dividing the soup evenly into two bowls, it is now ready to be served.

Nutritional Values (per serving):

Calories: 190 | Fat: 7g | Saturated Fat: 1g |
Cholesterol: 0mg | Sodium: 480mg |
Carbohydrates: 28g | Fiber: 3g | Sugar: 4g |
Protein: 3g

CARROT AND GINGER SOUP

Ingredients:

- 1 tbsp olive oil
- ½ cup chopped onion
- ½ cup chopped carrots
- ½ tsp minced fresh ginger
- 2 cups low-sodium vegetable broth
- ¼ tsp salt
- ¼ tsp black pepper

Instructions:

1. Heat the olive oil in a medium saucepan over medium heat. Cook the onion, carrots, and ginger in the pot for 4-5 minutes, stirring regularly, until the veggies are softened.
2. To the pot, add the vegetable broth, salt, and black pepper.
3. Bring the mixture to a boil when the veggies have softened. Reduce the heat to low and continue to cook the soup for 15-20 minutes, stirring periodically, until the carrots are soft.
4. Puree the soup with an immersion blender until it achieves a smooth consistency. When combining boiling liquids, use caution and wait for the soup to cool slightly before blending.
5. Evenly divide the pureed soup into two bowls and serve immediately. If preferred, top with fresh herbs or a splash of olive oil.

Nutritional Values (per serving):

Calories: 130 | Fat: 7g | Saturated Fat: 1g |
Cholesterol: 0mg | Sodium: 480mg |
Carbohydrates: 15g | Fiber: 3g | Sugar: 6g |
Protein: 2g

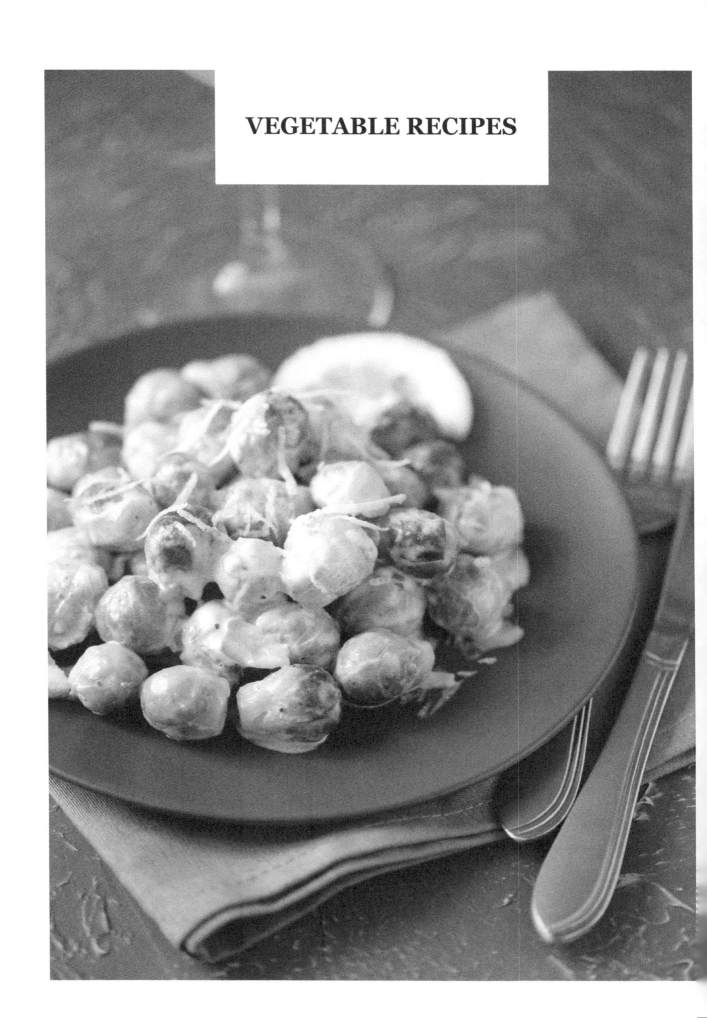

VEGETABLE RECIPES

GARLIC-ROASTED BRUSSELS SPROUTS

Ingredients:

- 2 cups Brussels sprouts, halved
- 1 tbsp olive oil
- 2 cloves garlic, minced
- ¼ tsp salt
- ¼ tsp black pepper

Instructions:

1. Turn the oven's temperature up to 400 °F (200 °C). Line a baking sheet with parchment paper.
2. In a bowl, combine Brussels sprouts, olive oil, garlic, salt, and pepper. Toss to coat evenly.
3. Place the Brussels sprouts in one layer on the ready-to-use baking tray.
4. Place the vegetables on a baking sheet and roast them in the oven for 20-25 minutes, or until they are tender and slightly crispy. Serve immediately.

Nutritional Values (per serving):

Calories: 100 | Fat: 7g | Saturated Fat: 1g | Cholesterol: 0mg | Sodium: 330mg | Carbohydrates: 8g | Fiber: 3g | Sugar: 2g | Protein: 3g

CAULIFLOWER FRIED RICE

Ingredients:

- 1 tbsp olive oil
- ½ cup chopped onion
- ½ cup chopped bell pepper
- ½ cup chopped carrots
- 2 cups cauliflower rice
- ¼ cup low-sodium soy sauce
- ¼ tsp black pepper

Instructions:

1. Warm the olive oil in a sizable frying pan on medium heat. Include the onion, bell pepper, and carrots. Sauté for around 5-7 minutes until the vegetables become tender.
2. Add the cauliflower rice, soy sauce, and black pepper. Add the cauliflower to the pot and continue cooking for another 5-7 minutes, stirring occasionally, until the cauliflower becomes soft.
3. Ladle the cauliflower fried rice into two plates and serve immediately.

Nutritional Values (per serving):

Calories: 180 | Fat: 7g | Saturated Fat: 1g | Cholesterol: 0mg | Sodium: 480mg | Carbohydrates: 25g | Fiber: 6g | Sugar: 9g | Protein: 7g

BALSAMIC GLAZED CARROTS

Ingredients:

- 2 cups baby carrots
- 1 tbsp olive oil
- 2 tbsp balsamic vinegar
- ½ tsp dried thyme
- ¼ tsp salt
- ¼ tsp black pepper

Instructions:

1. Set the oven's temperature to 425°F (220°C). Line a baking sheet with parchment paper.
2. In a bowl, combine baby carrots, olive oil, balsamic vinegar, thyme, salt, and pepper. Toss to coat evenly.
3. Arrange the carrots in a single layer on the prepared baking sheet.
4. Roast the carrots in the preheated oven for 20-25 minutes, or until they are tender and caramelized. Serve immediately.

Nutritional Values (per serving):

Calories: 130 | Fat: 7g | Saturated Fat: 1g | Cholesterol: 0mg | Sodium: 420mg | Carbohydrates: 16g | Fiber: 4g | Sugar: 10g | Protein: 1g

CURRIED CHICKPEA AND SPINACH

Ingredients:

- 1 tbsp olive oil
- ½ cup chopped onion
- 1 clove garlic, minced
- ½ tsp curry powder
- ½ tsp ground cumin
- ¼ tsp salt
- ¼ tsp black pepper
- 1 cup canned chickpeas, drained and rinsed
- 2 cups baby spinach

Instructions:

1. Warm the olive oil in a sizable pan on medium heat. Incorporate the onion and sauté for 5 minutes until it becomes tender.
2. Stir in the garlic, curry powder, cumin, salt, and black pepper. Cook for 1-2 minutes, until fragrant.
3. Add the chickpeas and spinach. Cook the spinach for 3-4 minutes, stirring occasionally, until it is wilted.
4. Divide the curried chickpea and spinach mixture between two plates and serve.

Nutritional Values (per serving):

Calories: 210 | Fat: 9g | Saturated Fat: 1g | Cholesterol: 0mg | Sodium: 530mg | Carbohydrates: 27g | Fiber: 7g | Sugar: 6g | Protein: 8g

STUFFED BELL PEPPERS

Ingredients:

- 2 bell peppers, halved and seeds removed
- ½ cup cooked quinoa
- ½ cup black beans, drained and rinsed
- ¼ cup corn
- ¼ cup salsa
- ¼ tsp ground cumin
- ¼ tsp chili powder
- ¼ tsp salt
- ¼ cup shredded cheddar cheese

Instructions:

1. Set the oven's temperature to 375°F (190°C). Place the cut-side-up bell pepper halves on a baking sheet.
2. In a bowl, combine the quinoa, black beans, corn, salsa, cumin, chili powder, and salt.
3. Fill each bell pepper half with the quinoa mixture and top with shredded cheese.
4. Bake the peppers and cheese together for approximately 25 to 30 minutes or until the peppers have softened.
5. Serve right away.

Nutritional Values (per serving):

Calories: 220 | Fat: 6g | Saturated Fat: 2g | Cholesterol: 10mg | Sodium: 520mg | Carbohydrates: 33g | Fiber: 8g | Sugar: 6g | Protein: 10g

SWEET POTATO AND BLACK BEAN HASH

Ingredients:

- 1 tbsp olive oil
- 1 large sweet potato, diced
- ½ cup chopped onion
- ½ cup black beans, drained and rinsed
- ¼ tsp ground cumin
- ¼ tsp paprika
- ¼ tsp salt
- ¼ tsp black pepper
- 2 cups baby spinach

Instructions:

1. Warm the olive oil in a sizable frying pan on medium heat. Add the sweet potato and onion to the skillet and cook for 10-12 minutes, stirring occasionally, until the sweet potato is tender.
2. Stir in the black beans, cumin, paprika, salt, and black pepper to the skillet. Cook for an additional 3-4 minutes.

Then, add the baby spinach to the skillet and cook for 2-3 minutes, stirring occasionally, until the spinach is wilted.

3. Divide the sweet potato and black bean hash between two plates and serve.

Nutritional Values (per serving):

Calories: 260 | Fat: 8g | Saturated Fat: 1g | Cholesterol: 0mg | Sodium: 490mg | Carbohydrates: 43g | Fiber: 11g | Sugar: 8g | Protein: 9g

LEMON-GARLIC GEREN BEANS

Ingredients:

- 2 cups green beans, trimmed
- 1 tbsp olive oil
- 2 cloves garlic, minced
- ¼ tsp salt
- ¼ tsp black pepper
- 1 tbsp lemon juice

Instructions:

1. Bring a pot of water to a boil over high heat.
2. Blanch the green beans in boiling water for 3-4 minutes, or until crisp-tender. Drain and set aside the beans.
3. Heat the olive oil in a skillet that has previously been heated to medium-high. Incorporate the garlic and simmer for about 1-2 minutes, or until aromatic.
4. Stir in the green beans, salt, and black pepper and cook for an additional 2-3 minutes, or until the dish is well heated.
5. Stir in the lemon juice and serve right away.

Nutritional Values (per serving):

Calories: 100 | Fat: 7g | Saturated Fat: 1g | Cholesterol: 0mg | Sodium: 300mg | Carbohydrates: 9g | Fiber: 3g | Sugar: 4g | Protein: 2g

SPICY ROASTED CAULIFLOWER

Ingredients:

- 2 cups cauliflower florets
- 1 tbsp olive oil
- ¼ tsp smoked paprika
- ¼ tsp cayenne pepper
- ¼ tsp salt
- ¼ tsp black pepper

Instructions:

1. Set the oven's temperature to 425°F (220°C). Prepare a baking sheet by lining it with parchment paper.
2. Combine the cauliflower florets, olive oil, smoked paprika, cayenne, salt, and black pepper in a bowl. Toss to coat evenly.
3. Arrange the cauliflower in a single layer on the prepared baking sheet.
4. Place the baking sheet with the cauliflower in the oven and roast for about 20-25 minutes until the florets become tender and develop a slightly charred appearance. Once done, serve immediately.

Nutritional Values (per serving):

Calories: 110 | Fat: 7g | Saturated Fat: 1g | Cholesterol: 0mg | Sodium: 330mg | Carbohydrates: 10g | Fiber: 4g | Sugar: 4g | Protein: 3g

STOVETOP RATATOUILLE

Ingredients:

- 1 tbsp olive oil
- ½ cup chopped onion
- ½ cup chopped bell pepper
- ½ cup chopped zucchini
- ½ cup chopped eggplant
- 1 cup canned diced tomatoes
- ¼ tsp dried basil
- ¼ tsp dried oregano
- ¼ tsp salt
- ¼ tsp black pepper

Instructions:

1. On medium heat, warm the olive oil in a large cooking pan. Add the onion, bell pepper, zucchini, and eggplant. Allow the vegetables to cook for approximately 7 to 8 minutes or until they have been softened.
2. Stir in the diced tomatoes, basil, oregano, salt, and black pepper. Bring the mixture to a simmer and continue cooking for an additional 15-20 minutes until the flavors have melded together and the vegetables have become tender.
3. Divide the ratatouille between two plates and serve.

Nutritional Values (per serving):

Calories: 150 | Fat: 7g | Saturated Fat: 1g | Cholesterol: 0mg | Sodium: 470mg | Carbohydrates: 20g | Fiber: 6g | Sugar: 10g | Protein: 4g

PARMESAN ROASTED BROCCOLI

Ingredients:

- 2 cups broccoli florets
- 1 tbsp olive oil
- ¼ tsp salt
- ¼ tsp black pepper
- ¼ cup grated Parmesan cheese

Instructions:

1. Set the oven's temperature to 400°F (200°C). Line a baking sheet with parchment paper.
2. In a bowl, combine the broccoli florets, olive oil, salt, and black pepper. Toss to coat evenly.
3. Spread out the broccoli evenly in a single layer on the baking sheet that has been prepared.
4. Place the broccoli in the oven and roast for approximately 15-20 minutes or until it has become tender and slightly crispy.
5. Take the roasted broccoli out of the oven and sprinkle a generous amount of

Parmesan cheese on top. Serve immediately.
6. Serve right away.

Nutritional Values (per serving):

Calories: 150 | Fat: 10g | Saturated Fat: 2g | Cholesterol: 5mg | Sodium: 480mg | Carbohydrates: 10g | Fiber: 4g | Sugar: 2g | Protein: 8g

GREEN BEANS ALMONDINE

Ingredients:

- 1 cup fresh green beans, trimmed
- 1 tbsp olive oil
- ¼ cup sliced almonds
- 1 small garlic clove, minced
- ¼ tsp salt
- ¼ tsp black pepper
- 1 tsp fresh lemon juice

Instructions:

1. Place the green beans in a steamer basket and steam for 5 to 7 minutes over boiling water, or until tender-crisp. Remove the steamer basket from the heat and set the green beans aside.
2. Heat the olive oil in a large skillet over medium heat. Cook the sliced almonds in the pan for 2-3 minutes, stirring regularly, until they are gently browned.
3. Add the chopped garlic to the pan and heat for another 30 seconds, or until the garlic turns aromatic.
4. Add the roasted almonds, steaming green beans, salt, and black pepper to the skillet. Cook for another two to three minutes, stirring constantly, until the dish is well heated.
5. Remove from the heat, drizzle with fresh lemon juice, and serve.

Nutritional Values (per serving):

Calories: 210 | Fat: 18g | Saturated Fat: 2g | Cholesterol: 0mg | Sodium: 300mg | Carbohydrates: 10g | Fiber: 4g | Sugar: 3g | Protein: 5g

GARLIC MASHED CAULIFLOWER

Ingredients:

- 2 cups cauliflower florets
- 1 tbsp unsalted butter
- 1 small garlic clove, minced
- ¼ tsp salt
- ¼ tsp black pepper
- 1 tbsp chopped chives (optional)

Instructions:

1. Steam the cauliflower florets in a steamer basket over boiling water for 8-10 minutes until tender.
2. Take a small saucepan and place it on a stove over medium-low heat. Add the butter to the saucepan and allow it to melt slowly. Put the minced garlic into the pan and cook for around 1-2 minutes or until it releases its aroma.
3. In a food processor, combine the steamed cauliflower, garlic-butter mixture, salt, and black pepper. Process until smooth and creamy.
4. Once the cauliflower is mashed to the desired consistency, transfer it to a serving bowl. If desired, garnish with chopped chives. Serve the dish immediately.

Nutritional Values (per serving):

Calories: 100 | Fat: 7g | Saturated Fat: 4g | Cholesterol: 15mg | Sodium: 320mg | Carbohydrates: 8g | Fiber: 3g | Sugar: 3g | Protein: 3g

SAUTÉED SPINACH WITH GARLIC

Ingredients:

- 1 tbsp olive oil
- 2 cups fresh spinach
- 1 small garlic clove, minced
- ¼ tsp salt
- ¼ tsp black pepper

Instructions:

1. On medium heat, warm the olive oil in a large cooking pan. Incorporate the chopped garlic into the pan and continue cooking for another 30 seconds or until the garlic becomes fragrant.
2. Add the spinach to the skillet and stir occasionally until it wilts. This should take about 2 to 3 minutes.
3. Season the dish with salt and black pepper according to taste. Serve immediately.

Nutritional Values (per serving):

Calories: 80 | Fat: 7g | Saturated Fat: 1g | Cholesterol: 0mg | Sodium: 330mg | Carbohydrates: 3g | Fiber: 1g | Sugar: 0g | Protein: 2g

SWEET AND SOUR RED CABBAGE

Ingredients:

- 2 cups thinly sliced red cabbage
- ½ small red onion, thinly sliced
- ¼ cup apple cider vinegar
- 1 tbsp olive oil
- 1 tbsp honey
- ¼ tsp salt
- ¼ tsp black pepper

Instructions:

1. Place a large skillet on a stove over medium heat and add the olive oil to it. Warm up the olive oil until it is heated through. Incorporate the red onion into the heated olive oil in the skillet. Cook the onion for 2-3 minutes or until it has been softened.
2. Add the red cabbage to the skillet with the softened red onion. Cook for 5-7 minutes while stirring occasionally until the cabbage has become softened.
3. Take a small bowl and whisk the apple cider vinegar, honey, salt, and black pepper together until they are well-combined. Pour the mixture over the

cabbage and cook for another 2 to 3 minutes, until everything is hot and mixed well.

4. Serve the sweet and sour red cabbage as a side dish.

Nutritional Values (per serving):

Calories: 110 | Fat: 7g | Saturated Fat: 1g | Cholesterol: 0mg | Sodium: 320mg | Carbohydrates: 13g | Fiber: 2g | Sugar: 10g | Protein: 1g

OVEN-ROASTED ROOT VEGETABLE

Ingredients:

- 1 medium carrot, peeled and chopped
- 1 medium parsnip, peeled and chopped
- 1 small beet, peeled and chopped
- 1 small turnip, peeled and chopped
- 2 tbsp olive oil
- ¼ tsp salt
- ¼ tsp black pepper
- ¼ tsp dried rosemary

Instructions:

1. Set the oven's temperature to 425°F (220°C). Line a baking sheet with parchment paper.
2. Take a large bowl and mix together the chopped carrot, parsnip, beet, and turnip. Lightly coat with olive oil, then season with salt, ground black pepper, and dried rosemary. Toss to coat the vegetables evenly.
3. Arrange the vegetables on the baking sheet that has been prepared, making sure to spread them out evenly and in a single layer. Roast for 25-30 minutes, occasionally stirring, until tender and golden brown.
4. Serve the oven-roasted root vegetables as a side dish.

Nutritional Values (per serving):

Calories: 200 | Fat: 14g | Saturated Fat: 2g | Cholesterol: 0mg | Sodium: 320mg | Carbohydrates

EGGPLANT PARMESAN STACKS

Ingredients:

- 1 medium eggplant, sliced into ½-inch rounds
- ½ cup whole wheat breadcrumbs
- ¼ cup grated Parmesan cheese
- ¼ tsp garlic powder
- ¼ tsp salt
- ¼ tsp black pepper
- 1 large egg, beaten
- ½ cup marinara sauce
- ½ cup shredded mozzarella cheese
- 1 tbsp chopped fresh basil

Instructions:

1. Preheat the oven to 375 degrees Fahrenheit (190 degrees Celsius). Using parchment paper, line a baking sheet.
2. Combine the breadcrumbs, Parmesan cheese, garlic powder, salt, and pepper in a small plate. Dip each eggplant slice in the beaten egg, then in the breadcrumb mixture until completely covered. Place the prepared baking sheet with the coated eggplant slices on top.
3. Arrange the oiled eggplant slices on a baking sheet and bake for 15-20 minutes, flipping once during the cooking time, until golden brown and tender.
4. Remove the eggplant slices from the oven and top each with a dollop of tomato sauce and some mozzarella cheese.
5. Return the eggplant slices, tomato sauce, and mozzarella cheese to the oven and bake for another 5 minutes, or until the cheese is thoroughly melted and slightly bubbling.
6. Decorate the eggplant Serve parmesan stacks with chopped fresh basil.

Nutritional Values (per serving):

Calories: 270 | Fat: 12g | Saturated Fat: 5g | Cholesterol: 75mg | Sodium: 840mg | Carbohydrates: 30g | Fiber: 7g | Sugar: 8g | Protein: 13g

CREAMY POLENTA WITH ROASTED VEGETABLES

Ingredients:

- 1 cup yellow cornmeal
- 4 cups vegetable broth
- ¼ cup grated Parmesan cheese
- ¼ cup heavy cream
- ¼ tsp salt
- ¼ tsp black pepper
- 2 cups assorted vegetables (e.g., zucchini, cherry tomatoes, bell peppers), chopped
- 2 tbsp olive oil
- ¼ tsp dried thyme
- ¼ tsp garlic powder

Instructions:

1. Preheat the oven to 425 degrees Fahrenheit (220 degrees Celsius). Using parchment paper, line a baking sheet.
2. Heat the vegetable broth in a large saucepan over medium heat. Warm the broth over high heat until it reaches a boil. Pour the cornmeal slowly into the boiling vegetable stock while whisking constantly to avoid lumps from forming. Reduce the heat to a low heat and cook for 20 to 25 minutes, stirring regularly, until the polenta has thickened and smoothed.
3. Add the Parmesan cheese, heavy cream, salt, and black pepper to taste. While making the vegetables, keep the polenta warm.
4. In a large mixing bowl, combine the chopped vegetables, olive oil, dried thyme, and garlic powder until equally covered.
5. Arrange the vegetables on the prepared baking sheet in a single layer to achieve uniform cooking.
6. Roast for 15-20 minutes, tossing periodically, until soft and golden brown.
7. Arrange the roasted vegetables on top of the creamy polenta. Serve right away.

Nutritional Values (per serving):

Calories: 410 | Fat: 22g | Saturated Fat: 8g | Cholesterol: 40mg | Sodium: 1010mg | Carbohydrates: 46g | Fiber: 6g | Sugar: 6g | Protein: 10g

STUFFED PORTOBELLO MUSHROOMS

Ingredients:

- 4 large portobello mushroom caps
- 2 tbsp olive oil
- ¼ tsp salt
- ¼ tsp black pepper
- ½ cup cooked quinoa
- ½ cup chopped spinach
- ¼ cup crumbled feta cheese
- ¼ cup chopped sun-dried tomatoes
- ¼ cup chopped fresh basil
- 1 tbsp balsamic vinegar

Instructions:

1. Set the oven's temperature to 375°F (190°C). Using parchment paper, line a baking sheet.
2. Clean the portobello mushroom caps by removing the gills and stems. Brush the mushroom caps with olive oil after salting and peppering them on both sides. Place the mushroom caps, gill-side up, on a baking sheet lined with parchment paper.
3. In a medium mixing bowl, add the cooked quinoa, spinach, feta cheese, sun-dried tomatoes, and basil. Combine thoroughly.
4. Fill each portobello mushroom cap with an equal amount of the quinoa mixture, gently pressing down to thoroughly fill the cap.
5. Bake the mushrooms for 15 to 20 minutes, or until the mushrooms are tender and the sauce is heated.
6. Drizzle the balsamic vinegar over the stuffed portobello mushrooms and serve.

Nutritional Values (per serving):

Calories: 240 | Fat: 15g | Saturated Fat: 4g | Cholesterol: 15mg | Sodium: 570mg |

Carbohydrates: 20g | Fiber: 4g | Sugar: 5g | Protein: 8g

ZUCCHINI FRITTERS

Ingredients:

- 2 cups grated zucchini
- ½ cup all-purpose flour
- ½ cup grated Parmesan cheese
- 1 large egg, beaten
- ¼ cup chopped green onion
- ¼ tsp salt
- ¼ tsp black pepper
- ¼ cup vegetable oil

Instructions:

1. Place the chopped zucchini in a clean dish towel. Squeeze and squeeze the zucchini in the towel to get rid of any extra moisture.
2. In a large mixing basin, combine the zucchini, flour, Parmesan cheese, egg, green onion, salt, and black pepper. Mix thoroughly to get a thick batter.
3. Melt the butter in a large skillet over medium heat, then add the vegetable oil. Warm the oil in a small saucepan. Fill the skillet with heaping spoonful of zucchini batter, flattening each fritter slightly with the back of a spoon.
4. Cook the zucchini fritters in the skillet for 3-4 minutes per side, or until golden brown and crisp. Place the zucchini fritters on a platter lined with paper towels once they have finished cooking. This will aid in the absorption of any extra oil.
5. Plate the zucchini fritters and top with your favorite dipping sauce.

Nutritional Values (per serving):

Calories: 260 | Fat: 18g | Saturated Fat: 4g | Cholesterol: 55mg | Sodium: 480mg | Carbohydrates: 16g | Fiber: 1g | Sugar: 2g | Protein: 9g

CHICKPEA AND VEGETABLE CURRY

Ingredients:

- 1 tbsp vegetable oil
- 1 medium onion, chopped
- 2 cloves garlic, minced
- 1 tbsp curry powder
- ¼ tsp ground turmeric
- ¼ tsp ground cumin
- ¼ tsp ground coriander
- ¼ tsp cayenne pepper
- 1 (15 oz) can chickpeas, drained and rinsed
- 1 (14.5 oz) can diced tomatoes
- 1 cup chopped zucchini
- 1 cup chopped bell peppers
- ½ cup coconut milk
- ½ cup vegetable broth
- ¼ tsp salt
- ¼ tsp black pepper
- ¼ cup chopped fresh cilantro

Instructions:

1. In a large skillet over medium heat, heat the vegetable oil. Place the onion and garlic in the warm skillet and sauté for 2-3 minutes, or until softened.
2. To the skillet, add the curry powder, turmeric, cumin, coriander, and cayenne pepper and whisk everything together. Cook the spices for 1 minute, or until aromatic.
3. Add the chickpeas, diced tomatoes, zucchini, bell peppers, coconut milk, vegetable broth, salt, and black pepper to the onion and garlic in the skillet. Bring the mixture to a boil by combining all of the ingredients. Reduce the heat to low and continue to cook for 20-25 minutes, or until the veggies are soft and the flavors have combined.
4. Add the cilantro and serve the chickpea and vegetable curry over rice or flatbread.

Nutritional Values (per serving):

Calories: 270 | Fat: 12g | Saturated Fat: 6g | Cholesterol: 0mg | Sodium: 790mg | Carbohydrates: 33g | Fiber: 8g | Sugar: 9g | Protein: 9g

DESSERT RECIPES

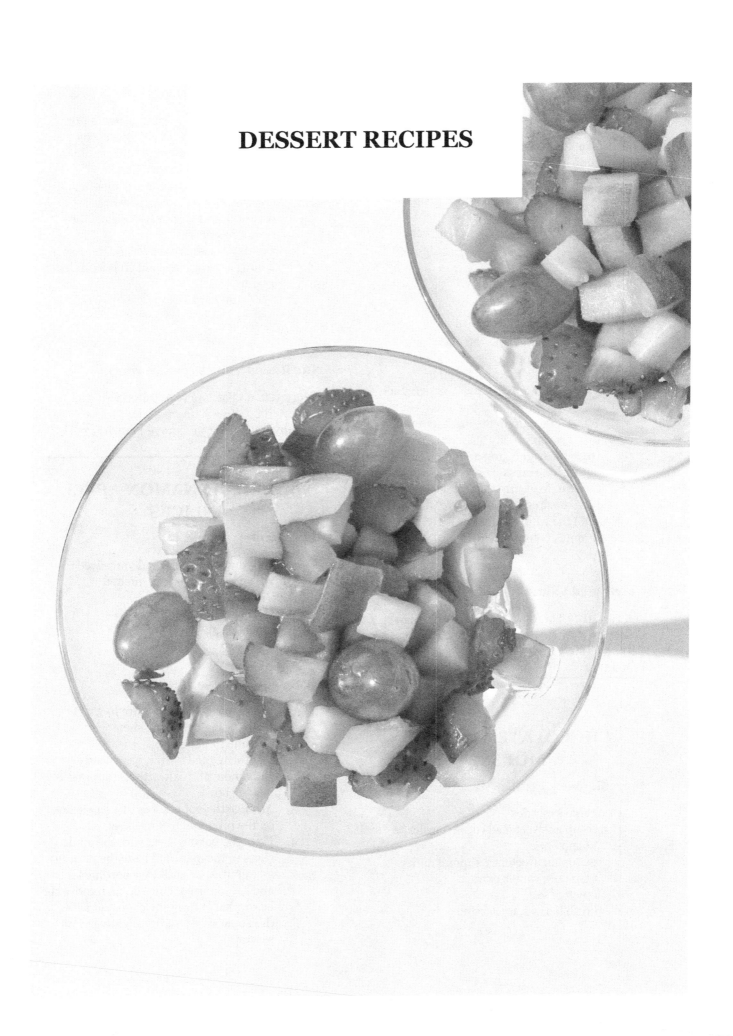

EASY FRUIT SALAD

Ingredients:

- 2 cups strawberries, hulled and halved
- 1 cup blueberries
- 1 cup raspberries
- 1 cup diced pineapple
- 1 cup diced kiwi
- 2 tbsp honey
- 1 tbsp fresh lime juice
- ¼ tsp lime zest

Instructions:

1. Put the strawberries, blueberries, raspberries, pineapple, and kiwi in a big bowl and mix them all together.
2. Take a small mixing bowl and combine the honey, lime juice, and lime zest. Whisk the ingredients together until they are thoroughly blended.
3. Once the fruit is prepared, pour the honey-lime dressing over it. Gently toss the fruit to ensure that it is evenly coated with the dressing.
4. Chill the fruit salad for at least 30 minutes before serving.

Nutritional Values (per serving):

Calories: 110 | Fat: 0.5g | Saturated Fat: 0g | Cholesterol: 0mg | Sodium: 5mg | Carbohydrates: 27g | Fiber: 4g | Sugar: 21g | Protein: 1g

CHOCOLATE AVOCADO MOUSSE

Ingredients:

- 2 ripe avocados
- ⅓ cup unsweetened cocoa powder
- ¼ cup honey
- ¼ cup unsweetened almond milk
- 1 tsp pure vanilla extract
- Pinch of salt
- Fresh berries, for serving

Instructions:

1. Put the avocado meat in a blender or food processor. Combine the cocoa powder, honey, almond milk, vanilla extract, and salt in a mixing bowl.
2. The ingredients should be smooth and creamy after blending, pausing occasionally to clean the sides of the blender as necessary.
3. Divide the chocolate avocado mousse among serving cups and chill for at least 1 hour.
4. Serve the mousse topped with fresh berries.

Nutritional Values (per serving):

Calories: 210 | Fat: 14g | Saturated Fat: 2g | Cholesterol: 0mg | Sodium: 50mg | Carbohydrates: 28g | Fiber: 7g | Sugar: 17g | Protein: 3g

BAKED CINNAMON APPLE SLICES

Ingredients:

- 4 medium apples, cored and sliced
- 2 tbsp unsalted butter, melted
- ¼ cup brown sugar
- ½ tsp ground cinnamon
- Pinch of salt

Instructions:

1. Set the oven's temperature to 375°F (190°C). Line a baking sheet with parchment paper.
2. Mix the melted butter, brown sugar, cinnamon, and salt with the apple slices in a big bowl.
3. Arrange the apple slices in a single layer on the prepared baking sheet.
4. Place the baking sheet with the apple slices in the oven and bake them for 20-25 minutes, or until they become tender and caramelized. Once done, remove the baking sheet from the oven and allow the apple slices to cool slightly before serving.

Nutritional Values (per serving):

Calories: 160 | Fat: 6g | Saturated Fat: 3.5g | Cholesterol: 15mg | Sodium: 35mg | Carbohydrates: 29g | Fiber: 4g | Sugar: 23g | Protein: 0g

COCONUT RICE PUDDING

Ingredients:

- ½ cup uncooked Arborio rice
- 1½ cups unsweetened coconut milk
- 1½ cups whole milk
- ¼ cup granulated sugar
- ¼ tsp salt
- ½ tsp pure vanilla extract
- ¼ tsp ground cinnamon
- ¼ cup unsweetened shredded coconut, toasted

Instructions:

1. In a medium saucepan, combine the Arborio rice, coconut milk, whole milk, granulated sugar, and salt. Place the mixture on a stove over medium heat and heat it until it begins to boil.
2. Lower the heat to a simmer and continue cooking the mixture, stirring occasionally, for approximately 35 to 40 minutes, until the rice is tender and the pudding has thickened.
3. After it has cooked, remove the pan from the heat source and blend in the vanilla extract and cinnamon powder, stirring until thoroughly combined.
4. Transfer the rice pudding to serving bowls and let cool for a few minutes. The pudding will become even thicker as it cools down.
5. Sprinkle the toasted shredded coconut over the rice pudding and serve warm or chilled.

Nutritional Values (per serving):

Calories: 280 | Fat: 13g | Saturated Fat: 10g | Cholesterol: 5mg | Sodium: 170mg | Carbohydrates: 36g | Fiber: 1g | Sugar: 19g | Protein: 5g

RASPBERRY LEMON SORBET

Ingredients:

- 3 cups fresh raspberries
- 1 cup granulated sugar
- 1 cup water
- ¼ cup fresh lemon juice
- 1 tsp lemon zest

Instructions:

1. In a blender or food processor, puree the raspberries until smooth. To remove any seeds, strain the purée through a fine mesh strainer. Set the purée aside once the seeds have been removed.
2. In a small pot, combine the sugar and water. Place the pot with the sugar and water combination over medium heat. Heat the liquid, stirring occasionally, until the sugar is completely dissolved. Remove the pot from the heat once the sugar has completely dissolved and let the syrup to cool to room temperature.
3. After the syrup has cooled, stir in the raspberry puree, lemon juice, and lemon zest. Stir the ingredients until it is completely blended. Transfer the mixture to an ice cream maker and freeze according to the manufacturer's directions.
4. Pour the sorbet into a jar with a tight-fitting cover. Place the container in the freezer for at least 4 hours, or until the sorbet has solidified.

Nutritional Values (per serving):

Calories: 110 | Fat: 0g | Saturated Fat: 0g | Cholesterol: 0mg | Sodium: 0mg | Carbohydrates: 28g | Fiber: 2g | Sugar: 25g | Protein: 0g

CHOCOLATE-DIPPED BANANA BITES

Ingredients:

- 2 large bananas, peeled and sliced into ½-inch thick rounds
- 1 cup semisweet chocolate chips
- 1 tbsp coconut oil
- ¼ cup chopped nuts or shredded coconut, for garnish (optional)

Instructions:

1. Place parchment paper on a baking pan. Arrange the banana slices on the prepared baking sheet in a single layer.
2. Place the chocolate chips and coconut oil in a microwave-safe bowl. Microwave the bowl containing the chocolate chips and coconut oil in 30-second increments. Between intervals, stir the mixture until the chocolate has melted and become smooth.
3. Dip each banana slice into the melted chocolate with a fork until completely coated. Shake off any excess chocolate before returning the dipped banana slice to the parchment paper.
4. Before the chocolate sets, sprinkle the chocolate-dipped banana slices with chopped almonds or shredded coconut if preferred.
5. Freeze the baking sheet with the chocolate-coated banana slices for at least 30 minutes, or until the chocolate has hardened. After that, place the banana bites in an airtight container and place them in the freezer.

Nutritional Values (per serving):

Calories: 130 | Fat: 7g | Saturated Fat: 4g | Cholesterol: 0mg | Sodium: 0mg | Carbohydrates: 18g | Fiber: 2g | Sugar: 12g | Protein: 1g

MINI FRUIT TARTS

Ingredients:

- 1 cup almond flour
- ¼ cup coconut oil melted
- 2 tbsp maple syrup
- 1 cup Greek yogurt
- ¼ cup honey
- 1 tsp pure vanilla extract
- 1 cup mixed fresh fruit (such as berries, kiwi, or diced peaches)

Instructions:

1. Set the oven's temperature to 350°F (175°C). Grease a 12-cup mini muffin tray with cooking spray.

2. Combine the almond flour, melted coconut oil, and maple syrup in a medium-sized mixing bowl. Combine the ingredients and mix until a crumbly dough forms.
3. Using your fingers, press the crumbly dough into the bottom and up the sides of each muffin cup to form a crust.
4. Place the muffin tin in the oven for 10-12 minutes, or until the crusts are golden brown. Remove the muffin tray from the oven once the crusts have done baking and allow the crusts to cool completely in the pan.
5. In a small mixing bowl, blend the Greek yogurt, honey, vanilla essence, and cinnamon until well incorporated.
6. Carefully remove the crusts from the pan once they have cooled. Fill each crust with a tablespoon of the yogurt mixture and top with a layer of fresh fruit.
7. You can serve the small fruit tarts right away or store them in the refrigerator until ready to serve.

Nutritional Values (per serving):

Calories: 150 | Fat: 10g | Saturated Fat: 4g | Cholesterol: 0mg | Sodium: 15mg | Carbohydrates: 14g | Fiber: 1g | Sugar: 11g | Protein: 3g

LEMON BLUEBERRY CHIA PUDDING

Ingredients:

- ¼ cup chia seeds
- 1 cup unsweetened almond milk
- ¼ cup fresh lemon juice
- 2 tbsp honey
- ½ tsp lemon zest
- 1 cup fresh blueberries

Instructions:

1. Combine the chia seeds, almond milk, lemon juice, honey, and lemon zest in a medium bowl. Whisk thoroughly until well blended.

2. Cover the bowl with a lid and put it in the fridge for at least 4 hours, or until the chia seeds have soaked up the liquid and the mixture has thickened.
3. Stir the chia pudding well and divide it among serving cups. Top with fresh blueberries and serve.

Nutritional Values (per serving):

Calories: 180 | Fat: 7g | Saturated Fat: 1g | Cholesterol: 0mg | Sodium: 65mg | Carbohydrates: 27g | Fiber: 7g | Sugar: 17g | Protein: 4g

STRAWBERRY BANANA SMOOTHIE BOWL

Ingredients:

- 1 cup frozen strawberries
- 1 medium banana, sliced and frozen
- ½ cup unsweetened almond milk
- ¼ cup Greek yogurt
- 1 tbsp honey
- Toppings: fresh fruit, granola, nuts, or seeds

Instructions:

1. Add frozen banana, almond milk, Greek yogurt, and honey to a blender or food processor. Blend the ingredients until they are smooth and creamy in consistency.
2. Once the smoothie has been blended to a creamy texture, transfer it to a bowl and arrange your preferred toppings over the surface. You can enjoy the smoothie immediately.

Nutritional Values (per serving):

Calories: 260 | Fat: 3g | Saturated Fat: 0g | Cholesterol: 5mg | Sodium: 115mg | Carbohydrates: 53g | Fiber: 6g | Sugar: 37g | Protein: 9g

MANGO COCONUT POPSICLES
Ingredients:

- 2 cups diced mango
- 1 cup unsweetened coconut milk
- ¼ cup honey
- ½ tsp pure vanilla extract
- Pinch of salt

Instructions:

1. In a mixer or food processor, mix the diced mango, coconut milk, honey, vanilla extract, and salt.
2. Blend until smooth and creamy.
3. Pour the mango mixture into the popsicle molds, making sure to leave a little room at the top for the mixture to grow.
4. Insert the sticks into the molds and then place the molds in the freezer for a minimum of 4 hours, or until the popsicles are thoroughly frozen.
5. Hold the molds of the frozen popsicles under warm running water for a few seconds to loosen them and remove the popsicles from the molds.

Nutritional Values (per serving):

Calories: 120 | Fat: 5g | Saturated Fat: 4g | Cholesterol: 0mg | Sodium: 40mg | Carbohydrates: 19g | Fiber: 1g | Sugar: 17g | Protein: 1g

PINEAPPLE COCONUT MACAROONS

Ingredients:

- 2 cups unsweetened shredded coconut
- ½ cup finely diced pineapple
- ⅓ cup granulated sugar
- ¼ cup all-purpose flour
- 2 large egg whites
- ½ tsp pure vanilla extract

Instructions:

1. Set the oven's temperature to 325°F (163°C). Line a baking sheet with parchment paper.
2. In a medium bowl, combine the shredded coconut, diced pineapple,

granulated sugar, and flour. Mix the egg whites and vanilla extract into the mixture and stir until well combined.

3. Scoop tablespoon-sized mounds of the coconut mixture onto the prepared baking sheet. Using your fingers, gently press the mounds together until they stick together.
4. Place the macaroons in the oven and bake for approximately 20 to 25 minutes, or until they turn a golden brown color.
5. Let the macaroons cool for 5 minutes on the baking sheet before putting them on a wire rack to cool fully.

Nutritional Values (per serving):

Calories: 90 | Fat: 5g | Saturated Fat: 4g | Cholesterol: 0mg | Sodium: 15mg | Carbohydrates: 11g | Fiber: 1g | Sugar: 9g | Protein: 1g

ALMOND APRICOT BITES

Ingredients:

- 1 cup dried apricots
- 1 cup almonds
- ¼ cup unsweetened shredded coconut
- 1 tbsp honey
- ¼ tsp ground cinnamon
- Pinch of salt

Instructions:

1. In a food processor, combine the dried apricots, almonds, shredded coconut, honey, cinnamon, and salt. Process until the mixture is finely chopped and sticks together when pressed.
2. Shape the dough into 1-inch balls and place them onto a baking sheet that has been lined with parchment paper.
3. After shaping the almond apricot mixture into bites, refrigerate them for at least 30 minutes or until they become firm. For storage, place them in an airtight jar in the fridge to prevent exposure to air.

Nutritional Values (per serving):

Calories: 100 | Fat: 6g | Saturated Fat: 1g | Cholesterol: 0mg | Sodium: 10mg | Carbohydrates: 11g | Fiber: 2g | Sugar: 8g | Protein: 2g

BAKED CINNAMON APPLES

Ingredients:

- 4 large apples, cored and sliced
- ¼ cup packed brown sugar
- ¼ cup old-fashioned oats
- ¼ cup all-purpose flour
- ½ tsp ground cinnamon
- ¼ tsp ground nutmeg
- ¼ cup unsalted butter softened

Instructions:

1. Set the oven's temperature to 350°F (175°C). Grease a 9x13-inch baking dish.
2. Set the apple slices in the baking dish you just made.
3. Combine brown sugar, oats, flour, cinnamon, and nutmeg in a medium-sized bowl. Use a fork or your fingertips to incorporate the melted butter until the mixture reaches a coarse crumb-like texture.
4. Sprinkle the crumb topping over the apples.
5. Once the mixture has been transferred to a baking dish, place it in the oven and bake for approximately 45 to 50 minutes, or until the apples are tender and the top has turned a golden brown.
6. Serve warm.

Nutritional Values (per serving):

Calories: 210 | Fat: 8g | Saturated Fat: 5g | Cholesterol: 20mg | Sodium: 0mg | Carbohydrates: 34g | Fiber: 4g | Sugar: 23g | Protein: 1g

FRUIT KABOBS WITH HONEY YOGURT DIP

Ingredients:

- 2 cups mixed fruit (such as strawberries, pineapple, kiwi, and grapes)
- 1 cup Greek yogurt
- 2 tbsp honey
- ¼ tsp pure vanilla extract
- ¼ tsp ground cinnamon

Instructions:

1. Thread the mixed fruit onto wooden skewers and arrange it on a platter.
2. In a small bowl, whisk together the Greek yogurt, honey, vanilla extract, and cinnamon until they are thoroughly combined. Serve the fruit kabobs with the honey yogurt dip on the side.

Nutritional Values (per serving):

Calories: 100 | Fat: 0g | Saturated Fat: 0g | Cholesterol: 0mg | Sodium: 20mg | Carbohydrates: 22g | Fiber: 2g | Sugar: 18g | Protein: 4g

DARK CHOCOLATE BARK WITH DRIED FRUIT AND NUTS

Ingredients:

- 8 oz dark chocolate, chopped
- ½ cup mixed dried fruit (such as cranberries, raisins, and chopped apricots)
- ½ cup mixed nuts (such as almonds, pistachios, and walnuts), chopped
- Pinch of sea salt

Instructions:

1. Place parchment paper on a baking pan.
2. In a microwave-safe bowl, heat the dark chocolate in 30-second increments, stirring after each, until smooth and melted.
3. Pour the melted chocolate onto the prepared baking sheet and spread it out in a thin, equal layer.
4. Evenly distribute the dried fruit and nuts over the chocolate. Press the contents into the chocolate with your fingertips until they are slightly submerged.
5. Once the toppings have been placed, place the chocolate bark in the refrigerator for at least 30 minutes, or until firm and set. After the chocolate bark has hardened, split it into smaller pieces and store it in an airtight container in the refrigerator for later eating.

Nutritional Values (per serving):

Calories: 160 | Fat: 10g | Saturated Fat: 4g | Cholesterol: 0mg | Sodium: 25mg | Carbohydrates: 18g | Fiber: 2g | Sugar: 12g | Protein: 2g

To receive your FREE eBook "The Anti-Inflammatory Cookbook" Scan this QR Code

COVERSION TABLES

Below are some basic conversion tables for the various units of measurement used in the recipes above. These conversions can be helpful when following a recipe or when scaling it up or down.

$425°F = (425 - 32) × 5/9 = 218.33°C ≈ 220°C$

VOLUME CONVERSION

1 teaspoon (tsp)	5 milliliters (ml)
1 teaspoon (tsp)	15 milliliters (ml)
1 teaspoon (tsp)	30 milliliters (ml)
1 cup	240 milliliters (ml)
1 pint (pt)	473 milliliters (ml)
1 quart (qt)	946 milliliters (ml)
1 gallon (gal)	3.785 liters (l)

WEIGHT CONVERSION

1 ounce (oz)	28.35 grams (g)
1 pound (lb)	453.59 grams (g)

LENGTH COVERSION

1 inch (in)	2.54 centimeters (cm)
1 foot (ft) = 12 inches (in)	30.48 centimeters (cm)

TEMPERATURE CONVERSION

Fahrenheit (°F) to Celsius (°C): (°F - 32) x 5/9 = °C
Celsius (°C) to Fahrenheit (°F): (°C x 9/5) + 32 = °F
Example Conversions:
$350°F = (350 - 32) × 5/9 = 176.67°C ≈ 175°C$

30 DAY MEAL PLAN

This 30-day meal plan provides you with a variety of breakfast, lunch, and dinner options, as well as snacks and desserts. Including a diverse selection of recipes in your diet can provide you with a variety of flavors and nutrients, promoting a well-rounded and delicious eating experience. It is important to keep in mind that adjusting portion sizes and ingredients to meet your individual dietary needs and preferences is crucial for maintaining a healthy and balanced diet. Combining all the recipes in this cookbook can make a 1900-day meal plan.

Day 1

Breakfast: Banana Oat Pancakes

Snack: Spicy Roasted Chickpeas

Lunch: Turkey Meatballs with Garlic-Roasted Brussels Sprouts

Snack: Apple Slices with Almond Butter

Dinner: Lemon Garlic Baked Cod with Green Beans Almondine

Dessert: Easy Fruit Salad

Day 2

Breakfast: Spinach and Mushroom Egg White Scramble

Snack: Greek Yogurt Ranch Dip with Veggies

Lunch: Pork Tenderloin with Balsamic Glaze and Cauliflower Fried Rice

Snack: Mini Caprese Skewers

Dinner: Spiced Lentil Soup with a Veggie and Hummus Wrap

Dessert: Chocolate Avocado Mousse

Day 3

Breakfast: Overnight Chia Pudding

Snack: Celery Sticks with Cream Cheese and Everything Bagel Seasoning

Lunch: Beef Stir-Fry with Broccoli and Balsamic Glazed Carrots

Snack: Avocado-Stuffed Cherry Tomatoes

Dinner: Shrimp and Veggie Stir-Fry with Curried Chickpea and Spinach

Dessert: Baked Cinnamon Apple Slices

Day 4

Breakfast: Avocado and Tomato Toast

Snack: Cucumber Slices with Hummus

Lunch: Baked Chicken Fajita Stuffed Peppers with Sweet Potato and Black Bean Hash

Snack: Ants on a Log

Dinner: Spinach and White Bean Soup with Lemon-Garlic Green Beans

Dessert: Coconut Rice Pudding

Day 5

Breakfast: Apple Cinnamon Quinoa Breakfast Bowl

Snack: Easy Edamame

Lunch: Greek-Style Grilled Chicken with Garlic Mashed Cauliflower

Snack: Peanut Butter and Chocolate Rice Cakes

Dinner: Pan-Seared Scallops with Garlic Spinach and Sautéed Spinach with Garlic

Dessert: Raspberry Lemon Sorbet

Day 6

Breakfast: Veggie and Egg Breakfast Burrito

Snack: Spinach and Artichoke Dip

Lunch: Balsamic-Glazed Pork Chops with Stovetop Ratatouille

Snack: Fruit Kabobs with Honey-Yogurt Drip

Dinner: Salmon with Dill Yogurt Sauce and Parmesan Roasted Broccoli

Dessert: Chocolate-Dipped Banana Bites

Day 7

Breakfast: Greek Yogurt and Berry Parfait

Snack: Sliced Turkey and Cheese Roll-Ups

Lunch: Beef and Vegetable Stir-Fry with Spicy Roasted Cauliflower

Snack: Popcorn with Nutritional Yeast

Dinner: Crab Cakes with Lemon Aioli and Oven-Roasted Root Vegetables

Dessert: Mini Fruit Tarts

Day 8

Breakfast: Peanut Butter and Banana Smoothie

Snack: Bell Pepper Nachos

Lunch: Slow Cooker Beef Stew with Green Beans Almondine

Snack: Veggie Pinwheels

Dinner: One-Pan Shrimp and Asparagus with Sweet and Sour Red Cabbage

Dessert: Lemon Blueberry Chia Pudding

Day 9

Breakfast: Vegetable Omelet

Snack: Frozen Yogurt Bark

Lunch: Sheet Pan Sausage and Vegetables with Garlic-Roasted Brussels Sprouts

Snack: Chocolate Banana Bites

Dinner: Baked Tilapia with Mediterranean Salsa and Sautéed Spinach with Garlic

Dessert: Strawberry Banana Smoothie Bowl

Day 10

Breakfast: Berry Oatmeal

Snack: Smoked Salmon and Cream Cheese Cucumber Bites

Lunch: Chicken and Rice Stuffed Bell Peppers with Curried Chickpea and Spinach

Snack: Cheese and Crackers

Dinner: Easy Clam Spaghetti with Stovetop Ratatouille

Dessert: Mango Coconut Popsicles

Day 11

Breakfast: Tropical Green Smoothie

Snack: Spicy Roasted Chickpeas

Lunch: Spaghetti Squash Bolognese with Balsamic Glazed Carrots

Snack: Apple Slices with Almond Butter

Dinner: Seared Ahi Tuna with Mango Salsa and Lemon-Garlic Green Beans

Dessert: Pineapple Coconut Macaroons

Day 12

Breakfast: Cottage Cheese and Fruit Bowl

Snack: Greek Yogurt Ranch Dip with Veggies

Lunch: Garlic Herb Pork Tenderloin with Cauliflower Fried Rice

Snack: Mini Caprese Skewers

Dinner: Seafood Paella with Garlic Mashed Cauliflower

Dessert: Almond Apricot Bites

Day 13

Breakfast: Multigrain Waffles with Fruit

Snack: Celery Sticks with Cream Cheese and Everything Bagel Seasoning

Lunch: Chicken and Broccoli Stir-Fry with Sweet Potato and Black Bean Hash

Snack: Avocado-Stuffed Cherry Tomatoes

Dinner: Baked Cod with Cherry Tomatoes and Olives with Parmesan Roasted Broccoli

Dessert: Baked Cinnamon Apples

Day 14

Breakfast: Almond Butter and Apple Rice Cakes

Snack: Cucumber Slices with Hummus

Lunch: Turkey Meatball Subs with Spicy Roasted Cauliflower

Snack: Ants on a Log

Dinner: Garlic Butter Scallops with Oven-Roasted Root Vegetables

Dessert: Fruit Kabobs with Honey Yogurt Dip

Day 15

Breakfast: Spinach, Tomato, and Mozzarella Frittata

Snack: Easy Edamame

Lunch: Grilled Portobello Mushroom Burgers with Stovetop Ratatouille

Snack: Peanut Butter and Chocolate Rice Cakes

Dinner: Lemon Herb Baked Salmon with Sautéed Spinach with Garlic

Dessert: Dark Chocolate Bark with Dried Fruit and Nuts

Day 16

Breakfast: Smoked Salmon and Avocado Rice Cake

Snack: Spinach and Artichoke Dip

Lunch: Greek Chicken Pita Pockets with Garlic-Roasted Brussels Sprouts

Snack: Fruit Kabobs with Honey-Yogurt Drip

Dinner: Spicy Cajun Shrimp Skillet with Green Beans Almondine

Dessert: Easy Fruit Salad

Day 17

Breakfast: Turkey Sausage and Veggie Scramble

Snack: Sliced Turkey and Cheese Roll-Ups

Lunch: Philly Cheesesteak Stuffed Peppers with Cauliflower Fried Rice

Snack: Popcorn with Nutritional Yeast

Dinner: Miso-Glazed Salmon with Curried Chickpea and Spinach

Dessert: Chocolate Avocado Mousse

Day 18

Breakfast: Chia Pudding with Fruit

Snack: Bell Pepper Nachos

Lunch: BBQ-Pulled Chicken Sandwiches with Balsamic Glazed Carrots

Snack: Veggie Pinwheels

Dinner: Shrimp Scampi with Sweet Potato and Black Bean Hash

Dessert: Baked Cinnamon Apple Slices

Day 19

Breakfast: Greek Yogurt with Granola and Berries

Snack: Frozen Yogurt Bark

Lunch: Beef and Vegetable-Stir Fry with Lemon-Garlic Green Beans

Snack: Chocolate Banana Bites

Dinner: Shrimp and Spinach Stuffed Portobello Mushrooms with Garlic Mashed Cauliflower

Dessert: Coconut Rice Pudding

Day 20

Breakfast: Avocado and Egg Toast

Snack: Smoked Salmon and Cream Cheese Cucumber Bites

Lunch: Balsamic Glazed Chicken with Stovetop Ratatouille

Snack: Cheese and Crackers

Dinner: Teriyaki Glazed Salmon with Parmesan Roasted Broccoli

Dessert: Raspberry Lemon Sorbet

Day 21

Breakfast: Pineapple, Banana, and Spinach Smoothie

Snack: Spicy Roasted Chickpeas

Lunch: Sausage, Peppers, and Onions Skillets with Curried Chickpea and Spinach

Snack: Apple Slices with Almond Butter

Dinner: Seafood-Stuffed Bell Peppers with Oven-Roasted Root Vegetables

Dessert: Chocolate-Dipped Banana Bites

Day 22

Breakfast: Quinoa and Berry Breakfast Bowl

Snack: Greek Yogurt Ranch Dip with Veggies

Lunch: Rosemary Lemon Pork Chops with Cauliflower Fried Rice

Snack: Mini Caprese Skewers

Dinner: Lemon Garlic Shrimp and Asparagus with Sweet Potato and Black Bean Hash

Dessert: Mini Fruit Tarts

Day 23

Breakfast: Green Detox Smoothie

Snack: Celery Sticks with Cream Cheese and Everything Bagel Seasoning

Lunch: Moroccan-Spiced Beef Stew with Garlic-Roasted Brussels Sprouts

Snack: Avocado-Stuffed Cherry Tomatoes

Dinner: Pesto Baked Scallops with Sautéed Spinach with Garlic

Dessert: Lemon Blueberry Chia Pudding

Day 24

Breakfast: Veggie and Hummus Wrap

Snack: Cucumber Slices with Hummus

Lunch: Spinach and Feta Stuffed Chicken Breasts with Spicy Roasted Cauliflower

Snack: Ants on a Log

Dinner: Tilapia with Lemon Caper Sauce and Parmesan Roasted Broccoli

Dessert: Strawberry Banana Smoothie Bowl

Day 25

Breakfast: Cottage Cheese and Fruit Bowl

Snack: Easy Edamame

Lunch: Asian Turkey Lettuce Wraps with Balsamic Glazed Carrots

Snack: Peanut Butter and Chocolate Rice Cakes

Dinner: Spicy Orange Glazed Shrimp with Oven-Roasted Root Vegetables

Dessert: Mango Coconut Popsicles

Day 26

Breakfast: Multigrain Waffles with Fruit

Snack: Spinach and Artichoke Dip

Lunch: Eggplant Parmesan Stacks with Curried Chickpea and Spinach

Snack: Fruit Kabobs with Honey-Yogurt Drip

Dinner: Poached Cod with Tomato Salsa and Garlic Mashed Cauliflower

Dessert: Pineapple Coconut Macaroons

Day 27

Breakfast: Almond Butter and Apple Rice Cakes

Snack: Sliced Turkey and Cheese Roll-Ups

Lunch: Creamy Polenta with Roasted Vegetables and Lemon-Garlic Green Beans

Snack: Popcorn with Nutritional Yeast

Dinner: Lobster and Corn Chowder with Stovetop Ratatouille

Dessert: Almond Apricot Bites

Day 28

Breakfast: Spinach, Tomato, and Mozzarella Frittata

Snack: Bell Pepper Nachos

Lunch: Stuffed Portobello Mushrooms with Sweet and Sour Red Cabbage

Snack: Veggie Pinwheels

Dinner: Zucchini Fritters with Chickpea and Vegetable Curry

Dessert: Baked Cinnamon Apples

Day 29

Breakfast: Smoked Salmon and Avocado Rice Cake

Snack: Frozen Yogurt Bark

Lunch: Stuffed Bell Peppers with Garlic Mashed Cauliflower

Snack: Cheese and Crackers

Dinner: Seafood Paella with Lemon-Garlic Green Beans

Dessert: Fruit Kabobs with Honey Yogurt Dip

Day 30

Breakfast: Turkey Sausage and Veggie Scramble

Snack: Chocolate Banana Bites

Lunch: Chicken and Rice Stuffed Bell Peppers with Garlic-Roasted Brussels Sprouts

Snack: Greek Yogurt Ranch Dip with Veggies

Dinner: Miso-Glazed Salmon with Green Beans Almondine

Dessert: Dark Chocolate Bark with Dried Fruit and Nuts

CONCLUSION

This book is your ultimate guide to adopting a healthier lifestyle, with a primary focus on heart health. This cookbook aims to empower you to create a diverse and flavorful diet that does not compromise your heart health by providing a customizable 30-day meal plan and a vast array of over 1500 delicious, low-sodium, and low-fat recipes.

Starting a heart-healthy journey can be intimidating at first, but this cookbook aims to make the transition easy and enjoyable. It takes you step by step through the fundamentals of heart-healthy eating and provides you with the tools and knowledge you need to create a sustainable and balanced diet. As you become more acquainted with heart-healthy ingredients and cooking techniques, you'll discover the joy of preparing nutritious and delicious meals for yourself and your family.

Adopting a holistic view of wellness is a critical component in maintaining a heart-healthy way of life. This includes making conscious, informed food choices as well as incorporating regular physical activity, stress management, and adequate sleep into your daily routine. Maintaining your health in all aspects will lay the groundwork for long-term success in preventing and managing heart disease.

Furthermore, the heart-healthy cookbook emphasizes the significance of developing a positive mindset and attitude toward your health journey. This approach encourages embarking on the journey with eagerness, inquisitiveness, and self-kindness, acknowledging that transformation takes time and that obstacles are an inherent part of growth. Celebrating your accomplishments while remaining open to learning and adaptation will result in an empowering and supportive environment that promotes long-term change.

As you delve deeper into heart-healthy cooking and experiment with different recipes and ingredients, you'll likely notice the numerous benefits of a heart-healthy lifestyle. The primary goal is, of course, improved cardiovascular health, but you'll also notice increased energy, improved mental clarity, and improved mood. Prioritizing your well-being is an investment in your overall quality of life, laying the groundwork for a healthier and happier future.

Having a sense of community and a support system is also important for living a heart-healthy lifestyle. Consider sharing your experiences, challenges, and successes with family and friends as you embark on your journey to better health. By involving others in your health journey, you will build a supportive network that can provide encouragement, advice, and motivation as needed. Furthermore, your commitment to a heart-healthy lifestyle may inspire others to pursue their well-being, resulting in a chain reaction of positive transformations within your social circle.

Remember to celebrate your accomplishments, remain open to growth, and share your experiences with others as you explore the world of heart-healthy cooking and embrace the journey to better health. You'll improve your personal health while also encouraging those around you to start their own journeys toward well-being. Here's to a lifetime of heart-healthy living and all the joys that comes with it!

Made in the USA
Las Vegas, NV
30 December 2023